NO LONGER PROPERTY OF
ANYTHINK LIBRARIES/
RANGEVIEW LIBRARY DISTRICT

Out in Time

OUT IN TIME

*The Public Lives of Gay Men from
Stonewall to the Queer Generation*

Perry N. Halkitis

OXFORD
UNIVERSITY PRESS

OXFORD
UNIVERSITY PRESS

Oxford University Press is a department of the University of Oxford. It furthers the University's objective of excellence in research, scholarship, and education by publishing worldwide. Oxford is a registered trade mark of Oxford University Press in the UK and certain other countries.

Published in the United States of America by Oxford University Press
198 Madison Avenue, New York, NY 10016, United States of America.

© Perry N. Halkitis 2019

All rights reserved. No part of this publication may be reproduced, stored in a retrieval system, or transmitted, in any form or by any means, without the prior permission in writing of Oxford University Press, or as expressly permitted by law, by license, or under terms agreed with the appropriate reproduction rights organization. Inquiries concerning reproduction outside the scope of the above should be sent to the Rights Department, Oxford University Press, at the address above.

You must not circulate this work in any other form
and you must impose this same condition on any acquirer.

CIP data is on file at the Library of Congress
ISBN 978–0–19–068660–4

9 8 7 6 5 4 3 2 1

Printed by Sheridan Books, Inc., United States of America

For George
who has shown me the true meaning of friendship since we were 4 years old.

CONTENTS

PREFACE

When I was growing up in the 1970s, in what was then a predominantly Greek immigrant enclave in Astoria, Queens, New York, my family and I often sat on our front porch during the warm days of summer, socializing with the other Greek Americans in our neighborhood. Each day at around 6 pm, two men quietly and sheepishly walked down the street past our front porch. The two of them went about their lives together, going to work, returning home, and walking by our house quickly, heads turned, perhaps in shame or perhaps fearing we would judge or mock them. More often than not, one of the men on our porch would comment "είναι τέτιος," a phrase in Greek that translates to "he is one of those"—little did they know, I was one of those too.

By 16 years old, it was clear to me that I was gay. At that time, as my sexuality was developing, so was my ability to detect members of my tribe. While working at my father's local community grocery store where I made deliveries, I realized two of our customers were a gay couple. One Saturday afternoon, one of the men phoned in an order, which I had to deliver. His instructions about the location of their apartment were clear—look for the house where his "friend," a particularly handsome man, would be gazing out the window on the second floor, likely smoking a cigarette. When I delivered the groceries to their home, I wanted nothing more than for them to tell me that what I was feeling was alright, but they too, like the men who passed by our home every day, rushed—in this case to get me out of their apartment, lest I figure out that they were together.

Neither of these couples appeared to be living openly as gay men who loved each other—at least not publicly. They could not marry; the government did not recognize their relationships; and their pride was squelched by the homophobia of our society, along with the ongoing perception of homosexuality as psychopathology, despite the rejection of this claim by the American Psychiatric Association—a perception that unfortunately resonates to this day.[1] I think of these men often and wonder where they are now, convinced that the community's worst enemy, AIDS, likely took their lives.

I've been much more fortunate, managing to navigate the treacherous waters of the AIDS epidemic as an openly gay man who came out in 1981 at age 18 during my first semester at Columbia University. When I disclosed my sexual identity to my parents, my father was calm and intellectual, as he was with all matters in his life, the same man who would come to my room every night while I was growing up to pick up a volume of the encyclopedia, which he would read in his bed. My mother, however, stuck in the 1950s Greek culture that she emigrated from, was tearful, blaming herself and believing that if I moved back home, I'd be "fine"—I told her no amount of chicken soup would do the trick. Over time she evolved and became nothing but loving and supportive, even offering some sound motherly advice on my wedding day when I married my husband Bobby.

When I was appointed Dean of the School of Public Health at Rutgers University, I loudly and proudly announced myself as an openly gay man, which ended up as a headline above the fold a of the school newspaper, *The Daily Targum*. I know other gay men have been in similar roles at Rutgers and in academia, but few, if any, have been so vociferous in being a higher education leader and a gay man. I led and lead with being gay. My actions in taking the position were part of an intentional messaging to all gay men, and to the LGBTQ population at large, that a man in his fifties, like me, who is openly gay, married, and speaks often of his husband Bobby, could in this day and age, at least in a blue state, achieve a high level of prominence, even in an institution of higher learning, which are often much less progressive than they are thought to be. Even for myself, this achievement was one I thought I would never realize, the child of Greek immigrants with sixth-grade educations, and believing I had reached the glass ceiling in my profession due to my sexual identity. But Rutgers proved me wrong and my colleagues took pride in this story—an experience that was far from those that I had had in the past.

I attribute my successful career to being comfortable inside my skin and working hard to make my way in the world away from where I felt misunderstood. I often joke if I had not been gay, I'd be a tradesman married to a Greek American woman living in some working-class neighborhood of Queens, New York. Though there's nothing wrong with that, I prefer how I have led my life and how it has developed throughout the years. So to me, being gay was a great gift and blessing from the gods.

Throughout my career I have studied and advocated for the health of gay men, particularly in regard to the interconnectedness of gay identity, substance use and abuse, and HIV. I have written extensively on these topics, along with many others revolving around the issues gay men deal with today and have dealt with in the past. In my most recent book, *The AIDS Generation*, I sought to add to the growing literature of LGBTQ history. Only now is our history—LGBTQ history—being written. It is my hope that all of my work can help contribute to this effort, just as the work of filmmaker David France whose documentary, *The Life and Death of Marsha P. Johnson* told the story of this pioneer activist whose death remains unsolved to this day, and like the memoir *When We Rise*, written by another activist and creator of the AIDS Memorial Quilt, Cleve Jones, which traces the evolution of the LGBTQ rights movement across the decades, from Stonewall, through AIDS, and beyond.

When I began researching and writing this book, the overriding goal was simple—to share the coming out stories of gay men across the generations. Though documenting our history is still at the core of this project, my aim was to also decipher changes and constants in the coming out experience across space and time. In depicting the ongoing struggles that we face, I have taken strides to dismiss notions that coming out is no longer a complex or difficult phenomenon. In truth, it is the very same phenomenon that it was in the 1950s. What differs is the landscape, the scenery; the psychological process one experiences and the feelings of otherness one begins to have at a very young age are no different today than they were in days gone by. What differs is the increasingly larger proportion of enlightened loving parents, like my own, whose son is not lesser in their eyes just because he's gay; he is still the little boy they have loved since birth.

Unfortunately, many people were not raised and loved by parents like mine, Niko and Kalliope, and the reality for LGBTQ individuals is far from ideal. In a 2013 Pew Research Center report[2] over 90% agreed that society was more accepting of LGBTQ individuals than it had been 10 years prior to the survey; still some 58% had been subject to slurs or jokes, 30% rejected by their families, and 30% threatened or physically attacked. Telling and relevant to this book, a mere half had disclosed their sexual or gender identities to their mothers and only some 40% to their fathers, further supporting the complexities of coming out even in this more "enlightened" era.

There is also still so much to be done in drawing connections between the challenges of coming out and the health of gay men, another issue at the center of this book. We have much for which to be grateful in close-to-four-decades since the first cases of AIDS were detected, but this disease continues to haunt us, and with no cure in sight, the challenge remains for our nation and the world. The work we undertake regarding the health of gay men in the United States must continue to evolve. It is no coincidence that gay men continue to experience health disparities—whether HIV, substance abuse, depression, or a myriad other problems—due to almost daily discrimination, in the form of macro- and microaggressions. Like any marginalized group, this situation takes its toll on our well-being. The health, of gay men is shaped significantly by life experiences, struggles to come out, and subtle, and not-so-subtle, bullying. So to improve our health, it is not enough to focus solely on behavior—we must attend to the social and structural inequalities and discrimination that shape our lives, including our coming out processes.

I have also found in my work that, too often, representations of gay men's lives are based on the experiences of white men, often white men of privilege, who have the means or vehicles to tell their stories. But these men do not represent the totality, and in fact, there is a wealth of knowledge to be gained from documenting and understanding the lives of a diverse set of gay cisgender men. In effect, this book is also informed by my determination to give voice to a variety of different men, not just across generations but also across race, culture, ethnicity, nation of birth, and socioeconomic status.

As important as any other driver for this book is my desire to demonstrate the resilience of gay men across generations. Much of the time, gay men's lives are defined by deficit, focusing on what we do wrong versus what we do right. In my talks and lectures throughout the country, I have noted that one way to think about drug use or sex risk among gay men is to focus on the minority who engage in these behaviors; another approach is to focus on the majority who do not engage in these behaviors. My point is that our overemphasis on deficit, which dominates the preponderance of academic literature—whether the topic be suicidal ideation, or HIV, or crystal meth use—is also responsible for perpetuating the negative depictions of gay men as sickly and villainous, much like the Hollywood imagery of gay men throughout the twentieth century, as is shown in Vito Russo's powerful book, *The Celluloid Closet*.

On October 11, 2016, I conducted the first interview for this book; coincidentally it also happened to be National Coming Out Day. As I began to write the manuscript, it was June 25, 2017, the culmination of Gay Pride week in New York City, ground zero for the fight for LBGTQ rights, and Pride Month throughout the world. It is remarkable to note that at the time this book was published, 2019 marks over a half century since the Stonewall Riots of 1969 in New York City, a demarcation point that defined, and continues to define, the lives of the LGBTQ population. This historic moment has shaped the life experiences of all the men with whom I spoke, regardless of the proximity of their birth to this historic juncture.

My great fortune as an academic is that I am provided the opportunity to work with and learn from those emerging public health scholars whom I am helping to train. The development of this volume from its inception to putting on its finishing touches was supported intellectually and emotionally in significant ways by three of these next-gen minds—Adrian Zongrone, Annie Ristuccia, and Kristen Krause. For their generosity of spirit and inspiration, I am forever grateful.

My hope is that this book, if even in a small way, will help continue this advancement, connecting us as a population of gay men across generations in time and place, while also shedding light on the work that still needs to be accomplished in the United States and abroad to push the LGBTQ movement forward. Every gay man whom I have come to know throughout the course of my life has experienced, and continues to experience, the process of coming out in an effort to live his individual truth. No matter our sexual background, race, ethnicity, or socioeconomic standing, we must all work together, providing emotional, cultural, and social support toward such efforts, ensuring the march toward full equality for the LGBTQ community over the next half century and beyond.

REFERENCES

1. Drescher J. Out of DSM: Depathologizing homosexuality. *Behavioral Sciences (Basel, Switzerland)*. 2015;5(4):565–575.
2. Taylor P. *A survey of LGBT Americans: Attitudes, experiences and values in changing times*. Washington, DC: Pew Research Center; 2013.

Introduction

Pride

It has been 50 years since a group of transgender, queer, gay, and lesbian individuals fought for their rights at Stonewall Inn in Greenwich Village, New York, physically, socially, and emotionally marking the onset of the gay rights movement. Since that time, much in US society has changed. In 1973, over 70% of Americans thought homosexuality was "always wrong," a figure that decreased to less than 50% in 2012.[1] By 2017, two years after the case of *Obergefell v. Hodges*, which created a national legal basis for marriage equality, 62% of Americans supported marriage in same-sex couples—74% among Millennials and 65% among Generation Xers.[2] Somewhat surprisingly, similar patterns have emerged among evangelical Christians.[3] Today, it appears that the lesbian, gay, bisexual, transgender, and queer (LGBTQ) community's place in American society is, at a minimum, beginning to be solidified.

Despite these promising trends in societal attitudes, many continue to spew hate at the LGBTQ community, including some political and religious figures, and there is a substantial portion of Americans who still demean, ridicule, victimize, attack, and even kill LGBTQ people. These macroaggressions, found throughout the United States, have been precipitated by responses to recent legal advances that have sought to protect LGBTQ rights, enhancing gay men's and women's well-being, health, and safety. In turn, state and local legislatures in conservative locales have enacted efforts to undermine these rights, including marriage equality, under the guise of religious freedom.

For example, Senator Roy Moore, a supposed faithful Christian who has been accused of sexually abusing young girls, has openly debased the lives of gay men and worked toward denying their rights.[4] Meanwhile, 2017 was the first year that NYC Pride was televised—though it's been a mainstay celebration and march in the city since 1970—but also the first time in many years that the White House failed to fully recognize Pride Month.

Twenty-seventeen was also the year of *Pidgeon v. Turner*, a case that the Supreme Court refused to hear, maintaining the lower Texas State Supreme Court's decision to deny spousal benefits to same-sex spouses of Texas state government employees, a decision that bigots heralded as "a Christmas gift."[5] This banner year further evoked the hate and ignorance of Ronald Reagan, when US president Donald Trump issued a World AIDS Day proclamation without a single utterance of the word "gay," nor any mention of the chaos this disease has created for the LGBTQ community.[6] Gay men also continue to be bombarded with venom like that of Mike Pence and other social conservatives whose targeted discrimination undermines LGBTQ rights and health.[7] During the 2017 Los Angeles Resist March, which replaced the Los Angeles Pride March in response to the endless barrage of hate by the presidential administration, conservative pundit Tomi Lahren referred to the event as a "crybaby fest of bullshit."[8]

These condemnations and slights are bad enough, but worse yet are the physical attacks perpetrated against LGBTQ individuals. The National Coalition of Antiviolence Programs[9] reported that the number of attacks on LGBTQ people rose from 1 every 13 days in 2016 to 1 every 6 days in 2017. Of the 33 hate crimes that had been committed in the first half of 2017, 12 were against cisgender gay men (gay men assigned the male gender at birth and who identify as male). And of course the horrific attack at the Pulse nightclub in Orlando is still fresh in the public's mind, heightening the fear for individual and collective safety for LGBTQ people throughout the nation.[10]

On the other end, microaggressions occur daily, whether at home or in places of work, coming from friends, family, and colleagues. These attacks are often subtle and veiled, but an attack is an attack—though they may be less obvious, they are just as insidious. I often think of a university professor colleague who insisted that being gay was a choice, not an identity—this person leads that school's diversity committee. Other microaggressions are sometimes less intentional, even stemming from a misguided attempt to support the LGBTQ community.

In this vein, traditional gay neighborhoods, or "gayborhoods," are being overrun by young heterosexual people who, in their zealousness to demonstrate acceptance, are not only "straightening" these environments[11] but also co-opting LGBTQ identities. This idea reached a crescendo when actor Andrew Garfield, during his run in the play *Angels in America*, stated, "I am a gay man right now just without the physical act—that's all"[12]—a statement both foolish and rude, despite his remarkable performance. I'm also reminded of a 2017 Pride event that I moderated at the LGBTQ Center of Hudson Valley, New York, where one young queer woman described the eagerness of her heterosexual friends, who identify as cisgender straight females, to attend Pride events to be "gay for the day." Though such actions might seem supportive to some, they are in fact hurtful and disrespectful, tone deaf to the issues and criticisms LGBTQ people must contend with every day.

In light of these circumstances, life as a gay man in the United States continues to be complex and multidimensional, shaped by a person's emotions, family, culture, religion, and society, structures that create the psychosocial burdens so many gay men experience. Notwithstanding the social and political advances that have created a better place for gay men in the United States, generation after generation must navigate and overcome hurdles while establishing their identities in a heterosexist world: for the Stonewall Generation it was the right to live their lives openly and freely; for the AIDS Generation it was the struggle to survive this deadly virus; and for the Queer Generation the battle rages on to make their place in a world filled with failure—such as the fallout from the 2008 financial crisis and growing income inequality—and to resist the monolithic, gender-rigid, racist perceptions that often permeate gay culture. Though these challenges are wide and varied, there is one that remains a constant for all generations of gay men, central to the battle for their existence: coming out.

MYRIAD IDENTITIES

In a 2017 article in the "Queer Voices" section of the *Huffington Post*,[13] James Michael Nichols depicts the powerful photographic exhibition on coming out by Alejandro Ibarra, demonstrating the universality of the coming out process as a rite of passage for gay men. What is often overlooked is that this rite of passage is a lifelong, continuous one. Gay men come out their entire lives and must fight for their place in the world in an effort to maintain and build their individual and collective dignity. For someone who is not part of the gay community, this condition of continually coming out may seem anathema and debilitating—and in fact it is. Yet coming out as gay men is what binds the community together, an emotional psychological process that defines so much of our lives and our struggles.

In the fall and winter of 2016–2017, 15 men shared their life stories with my research assistant, Adrian Zongrone, and me. We interviewed a nearly equal number of men from each of the three generations mentioned—the Stonewall Generation (men who came out in the late 1950s–1970s), the AIDS Generation (men who came out in the 1980s and 1990s), and the

Queer Generation (men who came out in the 2000s and 2010s)—which in many ways mirror the Baby Boomers, Generation X, and Millennial generations in terms of location in time, place, and cultural context. Though the interviewees' backgrounds and life experiences are diverse, they had all come out, however they defined "coming out," during adolescence or young adulthood. By situating the coming out experience during this period of life, the sociopolitical contexts of a given time period are similar across the men within each generation.

There are also commonalities that tie coming out experiences together across generations, whether you are a 78-year-old black man who grew up in Baltimore in the 1950s or a Chinese Mexican 19-year-old university student today, or anyone in between. While 59 years separates the generation of these two men, the battles they face continue, and both continue to resist the wars that are waged against them. Of course, differences exist as well, due to individual circumstances and personal experiences.

In telling their stories, each one of these men reveals who he is through personal narratives, which are key elements to the self-development of gay men, particularly gay teens. Autobiographical recollections provide an understanding of life experiences extending beyond the everyday mundane to reveal social and emotional paths. But their stories are not simply about the formation of one identity—a gay identity—although this was often the most prominent element of many of their narratives.

Instead, these narratives also show the multiple identities that these men have been developing throughout the course of their lives—as gay men, as lovers, as brothers, as sons, as professionals, in addition to their identities across culture, race, ethnicity, and location of birth, religion, and gender. The story of one's gay identity is not separate from the myriad other identities a person holds. These identities include that of the otherness created by a heteronormative society; the masculine or male identity imposed by the same society as well as the gay community; one's identity along the lines of race, ethnicity, and culture; the identity of drug use and partying; and one's identity as a sexual being who has sex with other men—this latter identity defining a great part of who we are.

SELF-REALIZATION AND AFFIRMATION—PRIDE

Disclosure of sexual orientation is an integral psychological component of getting to know oneself as gay. In sociologist Richard Troiden's model of sexual identity development,[14,15] the telling of others, known as commitment, is a critical element of this self-acceptance.[16] The idea is akin to psychologist Eli Coleman's conception of coming out[17] through an acknowledgment of same-sex feelings. The acts of self-acceptance and disclosure are also an essential step in gay identity development, as noted in Vivienne Cass's paradigm.[18,19]

Coming out as a psychological process—one where gay men have the need to announce, pronounce, and scream out their sexuality—is one that most people who are not gay do not quite understand. It's important to keep in mind that, unlike straight people, many gay men and women hold onto their feelings, hiding their identities, for years, as they are not bestowed the benefits of a society that just assumes all people have the same sexual orientation. Coming out also serves to remind others that members of the LGBTQ community are continuously trying to make sense of who they are and how they can work toward developing their own sense of pride and dignity as a community. This is to say coming out is an internalized complex process that only the person who is experiencing it understands; it is about the people coming out and not about those whom they need to tell. Said simply, coming out is necessary to realizing who we are—a phenomenon as crucial today as it was in the past. The act is a means of affirmation, a means of gay identity development, and an ultimate means to learn to develop pride in our own identities.

Through the stories in this book it is possible to more fully appreciate this notion of "pride" as central to the coming out experience. The meaning of the word has gained increased salience in my own life as I experienced the glee, honor, and respect with which these men shared their stories, even when there were events surrounding their identities that created troubling and sad circumstances. Not surprisingly, initial negative reactions to coming out may have a negative impact on well-being,[20,21] but they do not have to have a lifelong negative effect. The ability to embrace pride in oneself helps ameliorate the potential negative consequences that confront so many gay men in their coming out and everyday life experiences.

Throughout these stories, the sentence "I am gay" can be seen as a proxy for the sentence "I am proud of who I am." Perhaps this is the point of retelling coming out stories: to reaffirm one's identity and place in the world. For many of the interviewees, these conversations gave them an opportunity to further own their identity as a symbol of pride but also to affirm their deep-rooted belief that this identity was central and inseparable from who they are:

It's sort of like you're taking hold of your identity and that tattoo. I'm owning this identity. I'm a gay man. I've got a pink triangle on me—I'm gay. It means I can't take it off.

Wilson, the oldest of the men with whom I spoke, saw this pride in his gay identity as a powerful source of insight that may have not been bestowed on his life had he not been gay:

> And so, I'm grateful for that, you know—because I am able to, I feel, see a lot of things that would come—comes to me because of this perspective that I have, because of the sexual orientation that I have.

This sense of pride resonates throughout all of the stories in this book and underscores the narratives shared.

HEALTH

Concealing one's gay identity—and in effect squelching one's pride—is closely linked to aspects of diminished health. There is therefore a connection between coming out and the health of gay men. For example, evidence shows that a heightened HIV risk exists for men who have sex with other men but who do not identify as gay, or at least have not come to terms with their identities, a situation that may be mediated by the psychological distress associated with hiding one's sexual identity.[22] More recently, Ellen Riggle and her colleagues[23] have noted that higher levels of identity concealment are also associated with higher levels of depressive symptoms. Psychological well-being has consistently been associated with gay identity development and coming out,[24] and it has been suggested by Cass that pride in one's gay identity is a crucial element of a healthy self-conception.

Findings reported from the National AIDS Psychosocial Study[25] indicate that gay men who concealed their identities had a 3.2 times greater chance of developing cancer over a 5-year period than those who do not conceal their identities and approximately three times greater odds of developing other infectious diseases such as bronchitis, tuberculosis, and pneumonia. Despite some counterintuitive findings, it has also been noted that self-concealment is associated with substance use dependence among sexual minority men.[26] Such findings are consistent with literature that has shown an increase in physical health problems when psychosocial characteristics, such as gay identity, are concealed and in the psychological stress created by homophobia and discrimination within society.[27,28]

Coming out—self-actualizing, and integrating one's identity as a gay man—is likely to have beneficial impacts on the health of individuals and overall populations. Recently, the enactment of marriage equality has been linked to an increase in psychological health in the LGBTQ population.[29,30] In this light, legislation that protects the rights of sexual minorities and advances marriage equality may ultimately improve the health of gay men. Creating a society where gay men are safe and free to express their identities and their love will prove to be the greatest tool available in fighting the burdens of HIV and other sexually transmitted infections, substance use, and mental health states such as depression that undermine and diminish gay men's health. In other words, as a society, we must create circumstances that will ease the coming out of gay men; coming out will enhance pride, and this pride will improve one's health.

DIGNITY, EQUALITY, AND RESILIENCE

For gay men, the sociopolitical contexts of our world have changed, perhaps more so in the United States and western European countries than elsewhere. In countries such as Azerbaijan, Egypt, and Indonesia gay people continue to be arrested, as they were in pre-1969 United States;[31] in Chechnya gay men are placed in camps and killed;[32] and in Abu Dhabi HIV-positive gay men cannot enter the country, and when they seroconvert are deported. Still, this era in the United States remains charged with prejudice and hate toward the LGBTQ population. The challenge of coming out remains a very real one for many gay men, especially young ones whose socioeconomic and sociocultural backgrounds do not afford them the role models, support, or tools that would help them to further develop their gay identities, a reality that may be experienced more intensely for young gay men of color.

By facing these realities, however, all of us—gay and straight alike—can come to a better understanding of the issues our LGBTQ brothers and sisters continue to combat and how we are all implicit in the societal conceptions, constructs, and experiences of being gay in the twenty-first century. The stories I share in the coming pages are not rooted in the deficit models so many public health scholars espouse. Instead, they are rooted in a model of resilience. Like so many gay men who have come before us, and those who will thrive in the future, the men depicted in this book confront everyday challenges with determination. They willingly undertake the lifelong, and often exhausting, process of coming out, developing a sense of pride and living their lives with dignity. Consider the words uttered by 66-year-old Tom:

> I take great pride in being a gay man. I don't think that I would have had the success I've had, in life without being a gay man, and, the reason I say that is that if I had stayed where I was [rural Pennsylvania], I probably would be, if I were alive, I'd be fat, out of shape, with a wife I hated, and three kids, and I would be teaching

high school chemistry in Sunbury, Pennsylvania. Not a great future, not a great, not a great life. I also don't think my life would ever have been examined.

It is this self-awareness that all of the men with whom I spoke described many aspects of their lives—gay men living a life proudly and with human dignity are shown time and again throughout the pages of this book. And this life of equality, pride, and dignity is the life that we as gay men want to lead, deserve to lead, and must lead.

Without this sense of pride, we wouldn't have made such strides as individuals or as a community, nor would we be able to continue to do so in the generations to come. These individual narratives—detailing how gay men of the past and of today have had the strength to come into their own by coming out and the courage to lead their lives openly as gay men—help to define and illuminate the dynamics and conditions associated with coming out and being gay. As a population of gay men, we have much of which to be proud, and this is in no small part due to our fortitude, our grit, and our determination. These are the stories we should be telling, the stories of how, despite the odds, so many of us have made our place as contributing intelligent members of society, a trajectory attributable to our resilience and continuous fight to simply be who we are.

These are the stories shared in this book; these are our stories.

REFERENCES

1. Flores A. *National trends in public opinion on LGBT rights in the United States.* The Williams Institute; 2014.
2. Pew Research Center. *Changing attitudes on gay marriage.* Washington DC: Pew Research Center; 2015.
3. Bailey SP. Poll shows a dramatic generational divide in white evangelical attitudes on gay marriage. *Washington Post* 2017.
4. Jackson SC. Roy Moore blames "malicious" allegations on gays, liberals and socialists. *NBC News* 2017.
5. Carpenter D. How wrong was the Texas Supreme Court about equality for married gay couples? *Washington Post* 2017.
6. Gessen M. Trump marks a World AIDS Day without gays. *New Yorker* 2017.
7. Halkitis PN. Reframing HIV prevention for gay men in the United States. *Am Psychol.* 2010;65(8):752–763.
8. Michelson N. Twitter schools Tomi Lahren after she calls LGBTQ march "crybaby fest of bulls**t." *Huffington Post* 2017.
9. Waters E, Pham L, Convery C. *A crisis of hate: a report on homicides against lesbian, gay, bisexual and transgender people.* National Coalition of Anti-Violence Programs; 2018.

10. Stults CB, Kupprat SA, Krause KD, Kapadia F, Halkitis PN. Perceptions of safety among LGBTQ People following the 2016 Pulse nightclub shooting. *Psychol Sex Orientat Gend Divers.* 2017;4(3):251–256.

11. James S. There goes the gayborhood. *New York Times* 2017.

12. Cusumano K. Andrew Garfield, method actor, describes himself as a gay man while starring in Angels in America. *W* 2017.

13. Nichols JM. LGBTQ people share how they came out in powerful photo series. *Huffington Post* 2017.

14. Troiden RR. The formation of homosexual identities. *J Homosex.* 1989;17(1–2):43–73.

15. Troiden RR. Self, self-concept, identity, and homosexual identity: constructs in need of definition and differentiation. *J Homosex.* 1984;10(3–4):97–109.

16. Isay RA. *Becoming gay: The journey to self-acceptance.* Macmillan; 1997.

17. Coleman E. Developmental stages of the coming out process. *J Homosex.* 1981;7(2–3):31–43.

18. Cass VC. Homosexual identity: a concept in need of definition. *J Homosex.* 1983;9(2–3):105–126.

19. Cass VC. Homosexual identity formation: a theoretical model. *J Homosex.* 1979;4(3):219–235.

20. D'augelli AR. Mental health problems among lesbian, gay, and bisexual youths ages 14 to 21. *Clin Child Psychol Psychiatry.* 2002;7(3):433–456.

21. Juster RP, Smith NG, Ouellet E, Sindi S, Lupien SJ. Sexual orientation and disclosure in relation to psychiatric symptoms, diurnal cortisol, and allostatic load. *Psychosom Med.* 2013;75(2):103–116.

22. Rosario M, Hunter J, Maguen S, Gwadz M, Smith R. The coming-out process and its adaptational and health-related associations among gay, lesbian, and bisexual youths: stipulation and exploration of a model. *Am J Community Psychol.* 2001;29(1):133–160.

23. Riggle ED, Rostosky SS, Black WW, Rosenkrantz DE. Outness, concealment, and authenticity: associations with LGB individuals' psychological distress and well-being. *Psychol Sex Orientat Gend Divers.* 2017;4(1):54.

24. Corrigan P, Matthews A. Stigma and disclosure: implications for coming out of the closet. *J Ment Health.* 2003;12(3):235–248.

25. Cole SW, Kemeny ME, Taylor SE, Visscher BR. Elevated physical health risk among gay men who conceal their homosexual identity. *Health Psychol.* 1996;15(4):243–251.

26. Cortopassi AC, Starks TJ, Parsons JT, Wells BE. Self-concealment, ego depletion, and drug dependence among young sexual minority men who use substances. *Psychol Sex Orientat Gend Divers.* 2017;4(3):272.

27. Denton FN, Rostosky SS, Danner F. Stigma-related stressors, coping self-efficacy, and physical health in lesbian, gay, and bisexual individuals. *J Couns Psychol.* 2014;61(3):383–391.

28. Hatzenbuehler ML. How does sexual minority stigma "get under the skin"? A psychological mediation framework. *Psychol Bull.* 2009;135(5):707–730.

29. Raifman J, Moscoe E, Austin SB. Legalization of same-sex marriage and drop in adolescent suicide rates: association but not causation—reply. *JAMA Pediatr.* 2017;171(9):915–916.

30. Halkitis PN. Obama, marriage equality, and the health of gay men. *Am J Public Health.* 2012;102(9):1628–1629.

31. Cumming-Bruce N. U.N. officials condemn arrests of gays in Azerbaijan, Egypt and Indonesia. *New York Times* 2017.

32. Walker S. Victim of Chechnya's "gay purge" calls on Russia to investigate. *Guardian* 2017.

CHAPTER 1

Identities

Former New York City mayor David Dinkins understood the city he governed, from 1990 to 1993, as a beautiful mosaic. He used this apt metaphor to differentiate the city from others that were considered melting pots, in which identities were melded together, and sometimes lost, to create a whole. In a mosaic, all the individual elements are unique and beautiful, and though together they create a whole, the individual elements are never rejected—a metaphor that perhaps works well when envisioning gay men as both individuals and as a population. Gay men possess numerous roles and identities that do not meld into one, but instead collectively define the man. The ultimate goal of gay identity formation and development is consolidation—the integration of one's gay self with all other selves—the beautiful mosaic.

The development of this mosaic starts when we're quite young, even before we may have fully come to understand who we are. Growing up, those of us who were gay intuitively knew it, even when we didn't fully comprehend what it meant. This experience holds true across generations.

Take my husband Bobby's student Felix, whom Bobby met while teaching kindergarten. Felix arrived at school every day with beautifully coiffed hair and sporting a Prada bag. During class he would transform his workstation into a beauty salon or a Broadway stage, often working with the girls in his class. He was very attached to Bobby and would run to him whenever he saw him in the hallways. Felix knew there was something about Bobby he adored, even though he might not have been able to put his finger on it. He also knew that he himself was not like many of the other kids at school. He didn't know he was gay—but, in a way, he did.

Though Felix's story may seem stereotypical, it is very reminiscent of the emotional lives shared by the men interviewed throughout these chapters. From a young age, they all had a sense that they were not exactly like everyone else, and in the absence of gay role models, or their inability to perceive gay role models, their lives came to be defined by a feeling of being different, while searching to make sense of their identities. Even though social contexts have changed over the past 50 years, coming out remains integral to that search, and the accompanying emotions and challenges are fixed.

As people individually develop their own mosaic in relation to their gay and other identities, a collective mosaic is also created, one that is rich with all of life's experiences. Over time, different generations continue to add to this diverse community, helping this awe-inspiring mosaic grow in ways that may have never been expected or predicted. The 15 men interviewed for this book are a part of this whole, and just as their narratives are representative of their generation—whether Stonewall, AIDS, or Queer—their unique stories speak to their own individual search for identity and help create a better understanding of the coming out process.

THE STONEWALL GENERATION

The five members of the Stonewall Generation interviewed for this book range from age 62 to 78. Two of them are living with HIV. All five clearly and distinctly remember a period of time before the active and boisterous gay rights movement, when gay men were still being arrested for socializing in establishments such as the Stonewall Inn, now a National Historic Landmark. Reflecting on this time period, Tom, a 66-year-old white man, born and raised in a small rural central Pennsylvania town "on the border between the coal regions and farming country," stated,

> Look, we grew up in an age where who we are and how we expressed ourselves as sexual beings was abhorrent, you know, and for a long time, it was, you know, we were breaking the law.

The conditions and laws of the time fueled denial and the suppression of sexual identity, causing many gay men of the Stonewall Generation to never publicly come out.

Tom

Tom worked in the finance industry for much of his life but turned his attention to social work, earning his doctorate in 2017. He'd been supported and encouraged by his partner of 35 years, a psychiatrist, to pursue this new career. Tom's partner, Ben, had first entered this field in part because of the toll AIDS had taken on his community—something unfortunately common for members of the Stonewall Generation—and on his personal life including the death, in 1986, of Mark, a lover that he and Tom shared.

Similar to gay men of any generation, Tom's inclinations that he was gay began at a young age:

> Well, they started really almost from the time of my first memories, which, you know—I'll say they started around, you know, kindergarten, when I was five years old, where I realized something was different. Like, I couldn't, you know, couldn't articulate it; but I knew that it was, and that differentness grew.

That feeling grew more over the years. Tom's identity and destiny in life were linked, and he needed to escape the environment in which he was raised to realize what it meant to be a gay man.

> It means a lot of things but I suppose, at the core, it means my survival. I'm not sure I would be alive today if I were not a gay man. . . . So, the survival part has to do with escape. Getting away from a place that did not tolerate—back in the '50s and '60s when I was growing up—didn't tolerate queers. Uh, and if it was talked about at all, it was talked about in a hushed manner, of course.

In 1968, at 18 years old, Tom experienced the moment that so many gay men have when they finally understand the feelings that they have been harboring:

> Oh, there was a eureka—absolutely, there was a eureka moment. Absolutely. I was in college. It was the end of 1968. A good friend of mine, David—he was the person—the first person I ever had sex with—he had come down to visit me, and we were sitting in my parents' kitchen, and, you know, things got a little quiet, and he said to me, "Um, there's something I really want to tell you," and he said, "I'm gay." And, without ever having thought it, without ever having said it to myself, the first words out of my mouth were, "So am I."

Wilson

The sense of pride found in Tom's experience is also evident in the words of Wilson, a 78-year-old African American, HIV-positive man who grew up in Baltimore. Wilson's understanding of his place in the world as a gay man, even as a teenager, is reflected in his recollection of James Baldwin. Asked when he first realized that he might be gay, Wilson said,

> Well, the first thing that comes to mind is I remember an interview with James Baldwin on TV, because he was the big spokesman back in the dark ages, when we were going through "Black is beautiful." And he—he always smoked, and he—and this guy said to him, the interviewer said, "Well, Mr. Baldwin, what did you think when you discovered that you were a black gay male, and poor—black, gay, and poor?" And he puffed on his cigarette and said, "I thought I hit the jackpot." So, now at 78, I don't know if I hit the jackpot or not . . . But I do have a certain pride.

Despite this sense of pride, Wilson made it abundantly clear that he took no part in either the gay rights or civil rights movements of the 1960s. Speaking of one of his friends, a gay white man who lived in Greenwich Village in the '60s, when the Stonewall Riots took place, Wilson shared the following:

> He was living here in New York at the time, and was living in the Village, and was close to the Stonewall shit . . . it went on for about three or four days. And, like, the second day, he was—got in it, you know, and he joined [the] movement, and I said no way. . . . That was my other thing. I refused to be active in the civil rights. I said, I'm not carrying any signs. First of all, the sit-ins started. I was—I had finished high school, '56, I forget when the first sit-in was in North Carolina. . . . And I said I would never allow anybody to put a cigarette out in my head, to pour ketchup over my clothes, because those guys sat there and that's what the white people did, come a cigarette out in their head, and they had to sit there. I said no way I'd do it, because I'd kill him if he came, you know? If somebody poured ketchup on me, I'm not peaceful.

Ryan

For 62-year-old Ryan, his emergence as a gay man was defined by much more engagement than Wilson, or Tom, in the gay community, coming of age as a well-known and well-respected New York City drag queen. Ryan grew up in a northern New Jersey housing project in an Irish working-class family. "I didn't really have to come out," he said, "I was a screaming queen.

They knew." Ryan started doing drag around age 20 in a little bar in Newark, New Jersey, where his family had moved when he was 15, before emerging on the New York City scene. He reported, "I was the star of the Anvil," a notorious gay bar and sex club in what is now the banal and heterogentrified Meatpacking district of New York City.

Like so many of the men interviewed, Ryan describes his attraction to other men as taking place very early in his childhood: "Ever since I can remember. I always liked boys." Eventually this attraction would lead to an encounter in school that was the onset of Ryan's sexual life as a gay man:

> I grew up and—and I was like in the projects—and I guess I was in about fourth or fifth grade—I guess—sixth grade maybe? About fifth—fourth or fifth grade and I just—you know, I would be in the bathroom and I would see boys and be very attracted to penises. Well, one—one time, I guess I was about 10 or 11, a boy noticed I was looking at it. He says, "You want this?" And so—and I did. So, I gave him head.

Yet like so many of us, Ryan didn't connect his early sexual behavior or desires with being gay until his adolescence, when he had a life-alerting realization attributable to the theater:

> I was 15 years old and I was in Newark. I was out of the project. We were [living] in a house and the bus to New York City stopped right catty corner from my house. And mom and dad let me go into New York by myself. . . . My dad said. "When you get to Port Authority, go downstairs and there'll be a rack by where they sell the tickets [to musicals and plays] and there's "two-fors" . . . there used to be "two-fors" and you could go and get like half price or two for one and so I went to Port Authority, went downstairs, I found the rack. And I'm looking at all the—I didn't know what show I was gonna see because I didn't know what "two-fors" were gonna be there. So, I'm looking at all these "two-fors," Hello Dolly, Fiddler on the Roof, Man of La Mancha—no. I see one name and I went. I don't know why. I was totally clueless. I had no idea what it was about. So help me god. So, I took the "two-for" and I walked up to 54th Street to a little theater named Theater Four. Went there, gave them the two-for student ticket, $3.00, went into the theater, handed me the playbill, and the play—and it was a play. Not knowing at 15 years old it was an off Broadway show, not a Broadway show. And the play was the Boys in the Band. And there I am in the audience and I'm listening to it, and I'm listening to these men who I realize are homosexuals.

In 2018, *Boys in the Band* was revived at the Booth Theater in New York City by producer Ryan Murphy and starred numerous openly gay male actors, including Jim Parsons, Zach Quinto, Matt Bommer, and Andrew Rannells.

When the play originally opened in New York City on April 14, 1968, while several of the actors in the original production were gay men—such as Leonard Frey and Kenneth Nelson, both who have since died of AIDS-related complications—none of them were out. Still, Ryan recognized himself in the characters of the play:

> I had my Oprah aha moment. And I don't know—I mean—it was fate. I don't believe in coincidences. I believe everything happens for a reason. There's a—we never—may never know the reason, but there's some kind of circle or something that attracts us to certain things we're supposed to do in our lives and I guess that was one of them. . . . I'm watching this play and I'm realizing the gay characters and I'm realizing that I'm one of them, except younger.

Jim

Jim, now 66 years old, also began finding himself through theater. He became involved with the acting community in high school, a sharp contrast to his life at home. Describing himself as "symbolically Jewish," he grew up in a traditional household, conforming to his family's and culture's standards. The theater gave him an opportunity to meet other people outside his small world and feel more comfortable in his own skin. Jim's inklings about his sexuality, however, preceded his involvement in theater, also emerging when he was a boy:

> Being at the beach, and seeing guys who had their, you know, chest exposed, and their bodies, changing clothes. And I was wondering, "What the hell is my—why am I so fascinated with this?"

Jim began to realize and form his identity as a gay man in the 1970s and was shortly thereafter drafted to the Vietnam War. At the military screening he presented a letter from his psychiatrist that claimed him as "unfit for service" given his sexual identity. Though it may have been a difficult experience, being gay may have also saved his life.

Jim's sexuality and life as a gay man is defined almost entirely by his 41-year relationship with Joseph, the great love of his life and the first man with whom he had sex. Jim and Joseph met each other at a summer theater program in upstate New York, later marrying and adopting a son. After so many years together, suddenly, in 2012, Joseph died from a heart attack.

As a single father raising a now teenage son, Jim also had to begin facing the realities of dating, something he hadn't thought about for over four decades. Interestingly, Jim's identity as a gay man continues to be tied deeply to the life he made with Joseph, not specifically to "being gay":

> I'm proud, I'm out, and there are no hidden parts of me. But I don't identify, neces-sarily with that label. It doesn't because, it has to do with the sexual orientation, it has to do with maybe my way of looking at relationships.

Jason

In contrast to Jim, Jason's gay identity and much of his life story is based on his sexuality and sexual behavior. For Jason, the physicality of being a gay man is front and center, which is common for gay men when they first realize their sexual orientation, but continues to be central to Jason, who at the time of the interview was 67 years old. He's fond of referring to himself as a "short hairy Greek with a big dick."

A Greek American born in Massachusetts, Jason performed live sex shows on stage in gay theaters in the early 1980s and was involved in sex work during that time. He found both experiences liberating, enabling him to embrace his identity and reject the conservative world in which he was raised. When asked when he first started to identify as gay, Jason responded,

> It took a long time—a long time. I was having gay sex since I was a kid, um, but also straight sex. So, until I identified and said I was gay wasn't until the '80s. It wasn't until, like I started having sex onstage at the Show Palace. I guess I sort of identified as being gay, and it was very liberating, which we can talk about later, uh, but that was the first time I think. But then again, even then, depending on the job situations I had—one job, I was out; the other job, I wasn't.

Jason's understanding of his sexuality is also deeply rooted in his childhood fantasies of the 1950s:

> I was in love with Zorro. Did I know I was in love with Zorro—Guy Williams? No, I knew that I wanted to heal him, I wanted to fix his wounds, I wanted to—that kind of thing, and that's what I identified first.

The story that may best exemplify Jason is about his realization of his gay identity as a child and the lifelong linkage between his identity and sexual adventurism.

> They [his parents] would send me to my grandmother's in Pawtucket for vacation
> sometimes. I loved her; she was great. . . . I was the only Greek grandchild. The
> others were "xeni" [a termed used by Greek-Americans to describe non-Greeks]. So,
> I was the only one she could really talk to, even at 10 or 11. So, at 10 or 11, I'm going
> there—to Pawtucket—and, I'm walking around. It's a small town. My mother's
> side of the family had owned all these bootblack stores that were now candy stores,
> and she worked in them back in the '20s and '30s. So, I would go there, looking.
> They were all like—some were still bootblack, but some had magazines, and some
> had these nudist magazines and gym magazines, and they were the forerunners
> of all the gay magazines—the ones where, uh, there would be muscle-builders
> standing up with a beach ball in front of their crotch, and they'd be in the posing
> straps—all those things from the '50s. So, I was fascinated by that, and they would
> let me buy them. . . . I never brought them home. I threw them away. But the
> other thing about being gay in that time—which is why having sex onstage was so
> liberating, because it allowed gay men to really express themselves sexually without
> fear, without being humiliated. But, back in the day, when my mother would take
> me to dance school we'd go shopping, all the time. Shopping with my mother. So,
> we'd go to the Woolworth's, and I'd have to go to the bathroom, and there was a
> glory hole. Did I know what it was? I was so tiny and so short; I had to, like, jump
> up and hold onto the top of the thing to get up there. Um, and I didn't know. All
> I knew is somebody put their finger through, said—put it through, kind of thing.
> And so, I did it, and, uh, it felt good, and it was great, and boom! That was it. I re-
> member hanging on there, my mother screaming, "You done yet?"

THE AIDS GENERATION

Of the five men, ages 42 to 51, interviewed from the AIDS generation,
three of them, not surprisingly, are living with HIV. This proportion reflects
the epidemiological data for HIV infection among gay men in the United
States.[1] Analyses of these infection trends show that men born in the 1960s
were most impacted with HIV, the most deleterious effects on those born
between 1960 and 1964. Infection rates slowly declined in subsequent
periods, falling most dramatically among gay men born after 1975, who
would have reached emerging adulthood in or around the time of treatment
breakthrough in 1996.[1]

No one who came of age during the worst days of the AIDS epidemic
was spared the agony of this horrific disease. It didn't matter if you were
positive or negative; gay, straight, or bisexual; or where you stood along the
entire gender continuum, everyone was witness to, and many experienced
first hand, the tragedies and the resilience around AIDS that came to define
this generation. It is for this reason that so many of the individual identity
narratives of this group are often AIDS stories.

Emilio

Emilio's story is one of gay identity, HIV, substance use, and the related interconnections. For him, the notion of being a gay man is clear: "It means being authentic to my true self. That's what it means to me. My true self is a man who's physically, emotionally, spiritually, attracted to men." Raised in Spain to a father of Mexican ancestry, Emilio, now 51, came out to his parents in 1991 as both a gay man and HIV-positive through a letter, a copy of which he still has to this day:

> I actually have my coming out letter to my parents. I gave them the double whammy. Yeah. So I wrote this letter—first, I came out to my siblings one by one. I gave them phone calls. Then I wrote this letter to my parents, and I told them I would see them within three days and we could discuss things live and in person.

Many years earlier, Emilio had begun recognizing, and then developing, his gay identity:

> I think I knew at age 5 to be honest with you. My dad had these Playboy magazines in the basement. And I'd look at the magazines and I wouldn't care about the women. But in the back sometimes there were naked men, and I'd be like, **that's hot**. And definitely as a teenager, I used to jerk off to International Male and stuff like that. So, you know, I knew growing up.

Being gay did not seem like a safe or tolerable option in society for Emilio while he was growing up, so he often dated women throughout his formative years, as did so many of the men of the Stonewall and AIDS Generation.

> I met a girl in college at the Boston Conservatory of Music. We were dating, we got pretty serious, she met my parents, what not. I actually proposed to her, but she said, "No." Once that was done, the floodgates opened up. I started going to all the clubs. . . . I mean—unconsciously, I was trying to fight it for so long. I think once she said no, and I opened up and started going and really having open sex with men, that's when I felt like that's when it—I could say I was gay.

Seth

A 49-year-old HIV-positive man, Seth spent his formative years shuttling between New York City and Orange County, California, the homes of his divorced father and mother, respectively. A professional dancer for much of his young adult life, Seth, the youngest of three children, defines himself as a reformed Jew who drifted to "lesbian, feminist Wicca," eventually connecting with radical fairies, a global counterculture network that actively redefines Queer consciousness that some refer to as a form of modern paganism. Like many of the men of the generation after his, the Queer Generation, Seth spoke of being gay as one aspect of his interlocking and intersecting identities. Yet like the men of the Stonewall Generation, he spoke of his gay identity and the fulfillment of this identity with a sense of freedom and passion, emotion radiating from his eyes:

> What does it mean to be a gay man? Uh, all things considered, it means to be free—free of anything that's in the way of that . . . of my sexual identity, of my social—economic identity, of my spiritual identity, of my identity in relation to my peer group, to my colleagues, to my family. Um, yeah, it's so—it's such a web, interwoven threads, really.

For Seth, the sensibility of what eventually would become his gay identity was first apparent to him when he was 8 years old:

> Um, so let's see, my earliest memories, I think, um, being about eight years old, seeing the pictures of Jim Palmer in his Jockeys in the back of Cosmopolitan magazine and tearing, having tear sheets of him underneath my mattress. He was very tan. I look back at it now and it was like, mm, he's okay.

Lorenzo

Lorenzo, age 47, one of four children from the suburbs of New York City, in Nassau County, identifies as Italian American and was raised by a practicing and devout Catholic family. Like all of the men interviewed, Lorenzo describes the feelings he had during childhood that, though he didn't understand at the time, he would later recognize as part of the development of his gay identity:

> I remember watching an episode of F-Troop, and one of the Civil War soldiers, or whatever it was—the Union soldiers was staked to the ground by the Indians, and he was a blond boy, and I just remember going, "Oooh." He was literally staked to the ground with no shirt on, and I was like, "Wow." But I had known I was gay since I was a kid. You know, or at least not known I was gay, but the inclination was there.

Yet Lorenzo's fantasies would soon be overshadowed by traumatic sexual experiences as he was entering adolescence:

> My first sexual experience was kinda rough. My first sexual experiences—let me put that plural—were very rough. They were at the hands of a much older man. And I was way underage, like 12–13 years old. And I was more or less raped . . . two of them—two of them being Catholic priests and brothers.

A direct association has been shown between sexual victimization and risk taking in gay men,[2] and though Lorenzo grappled with both substance use and adventurous and risky sex for years after these harrowing experiences, he is now in a long-term relationship and relatively secure in his work and career. Still, neither of the men he spoke of were convicted, or even brought to trial, as is unfortunately too often the case for many men, often white and always with power. Much of Lorenzo's life experience as a gay man has been shaped by victimization and the inaction associated with the sexual assault he suffered as a child:

> He [the priest] was the—he was our eighth grade youth guidance guy, and I went to a parochial school and he somehow—I don't remember the exact circumstance of how he got me up to his room. I think it was—I wanna say it was—yeah, I do—I was riding my bike around town. I saw him outside, and he was friendly with all the kids. And I remember stopping and his saying, "Oh, come on up." And I remember going up, and the next thing I knew, he was not shy about what he had about in his room. Because at the time, your pornography wasn't confined to your iPad or your phone. It was stacks of magazines: Colt, and god knows what else. And, um, gay paraphernalia and toys, just out and about. And, you know, "What's that?" And the next thing I knew, he's telling me that, "Oh, I should get comfortable. Isn't it hot in here? You should take your clothes off." Next thing I know, he has me in my underwear, and I'm 13. And he's like, "Sex with a man is so much better. It's hard and rough and powerful. Not like soft and mushy with a woman." And I remember him grabbing my face, and squeezing my face and, like, my cheek, like my grand-mother or my aunt would've done. And without so much as a "Hello, how do you do?" I was bent over the bed, with his arm across my back, when he penetrated me. Um, that was—so, I kind of remember going home in a little bit of pain, con-sidering. "Wow, that happened," in my head. I didn't say anything right away to anybody, and I let him—he's like, "You know, obviously, this is our little secret." And then, it—I was there so frequently because he would, "Come over, come over, come over."

Due to his family's culture and community, along with the fear instilled by the priest, the actions continued:

[I was] afraid to say no because that's the culture I was brought up in: you listened to the authority, which was the priest. And this man used to go to everybody's house for dinner on, you know, Thursday nights he was at [this family]; Friday nights he was at [that family], and here, so forth. Um, and everybody held him in such high esteem because just the simple fact that he was a priest. And today's world, I think is—I'd like to think is a little different. I think—I'd like to think that we still look at them as being human, and really not the, you know, the god representation that we put on them. But back then, it was still. And they just did . . . [I kept going back] it was probably two reasons: one, when I finally was able to, uh, climax—because I was still young—it kinda felt—I was like, "Cool. That felt great." But, at the same time, he kept telling me, "Come back," and, "It's no big deal." And he said, "This is fine. It's the—you know—you and I. No one's gonna find out about it. And I'm, you know, you can't tell anybody." And basically, it wasn't a threat so much, but it was—it wasn't at least a—it wasn't a very verbal, uh, obvious threat. It was a veiled threat, if anything.

Huang

Huang, a 42-year-old HIV-negative man of Chinese descent, was also raised in a Catholic family, but he still struggles today with being an out gay man, even expressing concern that he might be identified in this book. (While I have taken precautions in protecting the identities of all the men, changing identifiable names, I was particular attentive to the story shared by Huang.) Huang's coming out story, like Jim's of the Stonewall Generation, is very much tied to the great love of his life, Peter, who had died only a few years before our interview, leaving Huang on his own, an older man looking for romance, kinship, and sex in the age of Grindr—no easy feat for members of the pre-"hookup app" era.

The notion of intersectional identities resounded clearly in Huang's response when asked what being gay meant to him:

I think it's just, like another part of who I am as a person. It's like a self-identifier so to speak. I'm not just only gay, I have other labels. I'm Asian American. . . . I'm male. I'm an uncle. I'm a stepfather. I, you know, there's a lot of titles of who I am, but it's part of who I am. So, it's not like the only thing that I am.

The pain Huang felt at the loss of his partner was palpable, Peter having only recently and suddenly passed away. They had built a life together with Huang helping Peter raise his three children from a previous marriage to a woman, all of whom are now adults and with whom Huang attempts to maintain relationships.

Yet Huang also demonstrated a sense of lightness in his storytelling, especially when describing his first sense of being gay as a young boy in elementary school:

> I always kind of knew that I was not straight, in the sense that like when I was a little kid in grammar school I had a crush, I mean, looking back now I think it was definitely a crush on my best friend at the time. And it was a he and I always wanted to hang out with him. And like really hang out with him and play a lot, but I had these different types of feelings or attractions, so to speak, and it wasn't toward a girl. . . . I wanted to hold his hand. I wanted to feel his face. I wanted to play with him. You know, like, he was the most popular boy in the entire class. You know, and there was any reason because he was probably the best looking guy in the class as well. And, I mean, looking back at it is kind of funny thinking about it, but back then I was kind of like a little, like, I knew I was not necessarily the right thing because I was raised Catholic as well.

Huang's challenge negotiating his identity remains informed by his upbringing in a strict Catholic home that was also rooted in Chinese culture, tradition, and values. For those of us raised in immigrant families, the message about the underlying "point" of marriage—procreation—was very real. Many immigrants' lesbian, gay, bisexual, transgender, and queer (LGBTQ) children, including most Greek and Chinese American gay men, wrestle with the pain of navigating their sexuality while trying to adhere to the tenets of their culture.

Immigrants in the United States tend to hold on to the values of the homeland at the time they emigrated[3] even if the values within the country they came from have evolved over the years. For example, many Greek Americans, including my own cousins, continue to maintain traditional often intractable and intolerant beliefs rooted in the Church while a large number of Greeks have progressed and Greece has morphed into a modern society. This sense of tradition and intolerance has always been central for Huang, even when he was young:

> And I know that my mom, at an early age, had already said things like, "Oh, when you get married, and when you bring home a girl, make sure the girl is Chinese and not, you know, white, or black, or anything else." And I'm like, little did I know, ten years later that well, it's not even gonna be a girl that I'm bringing home.

Stephanos

Also born into an immigrant family, 42-year-old Stephanos grew up in Hudson Valley, New York. His father was Greek, and owned a diner, and his mother was Polish. Describing his first inclinations of being gay Stephanos said,

> I remember like watching Batman the TV show, or like I had these Star Wars sheets, I remember—obviously I was vaguely turned on whenever Robin was like tied up for some—or needed saving, put it that way. And then, I remember always going to sleep and looking at Luke Skywalker on my sheets and wishing he was my brother. That was the thought, there's nothing really sexual add water—you know what I mean? Like, he was just like—I wanted a brother like to take care of me kind of thing.

Stephanos desire to connect with others with whom he felt a kinship may in part explain a feeling of difference or otherness that so many gay men sense but fail to understand as young boys. It's not surprising that this connection was found in the form of homoerotic imagery, as in the case of Batman and Robin, and the stories of outsider superheroes, like the mutants in the X-Men comic series. In fact, superhero mythology resonates with gay boys no matter their generation, normally permeating into their adult lives. The X-Men series in particular has resonance for LGBTQ individuals in its depiction of a group that is stigmatized by society but ultimately heroic (CITE) like so many sexual minority individuals. The X-Men character Iceman even recently came out in his mythology, searching to reconcile his identity from his past with his identity as gay, trying to maintain elements of both[4]—this too is our path as we emerge from boyhood to adulthood as gay men.

In time, Stephanos's desires were redirected from fantastical, fictional characters to other young men within his social circle, though his feelings were still unclear in relation to his gay identity:

> Like, so because I remember just always thinking like there was this gay guy when I was growing up. And, he was gay and every called—said he was gay and he acted very gay, and he was a waiter at my—at my uncle's restaurant, and I was like oh not him like you know although I had become aware that I liked other guys. But, I thought it was because I didn't have a brother at the time.

THE QUEER GENERATION

The men interviewed from the Queer Generation, ages 19 to 29, were the most foreign to me in that their life experiences emerged long after I was solidly rooted in my own identity as a gay man—chronologically, I could have been their father. Not surprisingly, given that the United States population of their generation is much more diverse than earlier ones,[5] these five men were the most racially and ethnically diverse of those interviewed. As a group, they also have higher levels of educational attainment than either the AIDS or Stonewall generations (i.e., Boomers and Xers)—a condition that became abundantly clear in their lucid and thoughtful, but often overly rational, responses to the questions posed. These overly-cognitive approaches to their life stories were indicative that these young men were still actively integrating their gay identity with other aspects of their being. Their intellectual thought process was matched by a clearly defined comprehension of contemporary social justice issues. Their diversity and level of education likely serve as the source for their deep-rooted understanding of intersectional identities, the struggle of gay men of color, and the progressive attitudes toward gender fluidity.

Gender fluidity is the representation and understanding that identity does not neatly exist in boxes or binaries but on a continuum.[6] This concept is not a novel one. Scientist Alfred Kinsey and his colleagues[7] understood this idea as early as the mid-20th century when they developed a scale to assess sexual orientation ranging from 0 (exclusively heterosexual) to 6 (exclusively homosexual). It is this very fluidity that has led to the use of the term "Queer" and why I have chosen to call this group the Queer Generation. Although some older individuals have taken offense to the term,[8] its use represents yet another step in the evolution of gay identity from the clinical, behaviorally focused, and society-imposed "homosexual" (pre-1959–1960s) to "gay" (1970s–1990s) and "queer," which are our own empowering terms linked to identity and not simply behavior.

The Queer Generation's fluid sensibility and intellectual grounding goes hand in hand with more expansive views of coming out and sexual identity development. San Francisco State University professor Michele Eliason[9] argues that most theories tend to "minoritize" sexual identity and that a more expansive view of sexual identity development would nest this identity in relation to others, including one's race, ethnicity, and class. I would expand this idea to include nation of birth and immigration status, culture, language, religion, and gender, in so much as everyone possesses intersectional identities that constitute who they are, as shown so pointedly in these men's stories.

Reid

No one interviewee exemplifies the characteristics of the Queer Generation more so than Reid: HIV-negative, 29 years old, born in Korea, and adopted and raised by parents from the Midwest. Reid's narrative is heavily influenced by racist experiences both within the gay population and US society at large. It's no surprise that when asked about fostering his gay identity, he focused on matters of race:

> I don't know that being gay was always a part of my identity, because I think, as the East and the West Coasts were slowly starting to accept gay people and to mainstream everything, the Midwest [was] going into that segue as I was coming out. I think that me being Asian was a bigger deal than me being gay, to be honest with you.

Reid often attacks the hegemonic white masculinity that typically defines the gay population, and like many men within the Queer Generation, he is adamant that he not be viewed as a stereotypical man. Having built a substantial social media following, he often uses his platform to bring attention to gay men who adhere to hypermasculine, white privileged norms and who dominate places like Fire Island Pines, a popular summer hideaway for gay men. Reid has experienced racism, body shaming, and simple intolerance in such settings and is fed up with the racist, masculine discriminatory culture within the gay community. This notion was exemplified in one of his Facebook posts: "I wore heels out tonight and I haven't felt so empowered in a long time."

Like all of the men interviewed, his sensibility of being gay was evident throughout his life, but his understanding of his attraction was informed by a fluidity in his identity:

> I think it was just always a thing. I was always just drawn to whatever I felt I was drawn to, and that happened to be men.

Miguel

Miguel, a 28-year-old man of Guatemalan descent, who was born to immigrant parents and grew up in the Boston area, shared similar sensibilities with Reid about identity and race. Miguel holds a more fluid conception of gay identity than members of earlier generations, and he is well versed in the terminology of gender identity:

> The person or people who I choose to fall in love with tend to be men or cis-identified men. I mean, I don't feel like I really fit in as a queer person because I feel like the identity of being queer is predominantly something that other people need. Visibly

queer people, trans people, people who exist outside of the binary—they tend to need that word, and I don't really need to—I don't really fall into that category. So I just identify as gay.

Miguel makes it clear that his gay identity is not the only facet of who he is, noting, "I knew that, like, I knew that I was gay, but I also knew that I was a whole bunch of other things too." Despite this more fluid and all-encompassing perspective of what it means to be a gay man, Miguel also sensed that he had an attraction to men at a young age including superheroes, though not Batman, X-Men, or any of the other characters that formed the basis of fantasies of gay men from earlier generations. "I really liked the blue Power Ranger for some reason when I was growing up. He [the actor who played the blue Power Ranger] was gay."

Though Miguel defines himself as a gay man beyond simple same-sex attraction and in more intellectual and broader terms, he still experienced many of the same uncertainties common to all gay men. He shared the following when asked when he first knew he was gay:

I didn't think about [it] like that. I didn't think like that in those terms. I think, I think I had an affinity toward hanging out with certain men for reasons that I was, like, looking for camaraderie. I was looking for friendship. But I was constantly looking. . . . I remember I went to summer camp one year, and there were, like, these two camp counselors that I just really liked spending time with. I didn't know why I liked spending time with them. . . . I was like seven or eight, yeah. I just really liked spending time with them. They were—but they were like—I don't know why. They were just nerdy and, and somehow I felt, like, connected to them, like, but I couldn't figure out why. I didn't know if they were gay or not at the time. I don't think they ever said anything.

These feelings were also evident to him at an even younger age:

Even before that, I used to go to a kindergarten . . . it was a bilingual school, so for like kids who spoke Spanish and English. And, there was a guy that I remember there, um, his name was Dean. Um, and I really liked hanging out with this kid, this guy too. He was, like, uh, really active like person who I—in my memory I remember him just constantly playing with us and being really, like, supportive of like—he was a, he was a great, like, teacher, like as a kindergarten teacher. I can still see him in my head. But, there was a year where I went to school and he wasn't there anymore. Um, I would find out later, as I got older that he was kicked out of the school because they found out he was gay. So this was in the '90s. He lost his job because, you know, they—obviously there was this assumption that because if you were gay working with children you must, you must have been a pedophile.

Yasar

Yasar is easy to remember clearly because of his beautiful nails, polished with a luminescent yellow. Ghanaian American, he was born in Greensboro, North Carolina, where he had a religious upbringing. The Ghanaian American church community and his physically abusive father shaped many of his early life experiences. Just as the men of his generation make sense of their sexuality beyond the sole indicator of male-to-male sexual behavior, Yasar describes the complex synergies of sexual identity, race, ethnicity, culture, and class that define one's identity. He also draws distinctions between the terms LGBTQ and QTPOC (queer transgender people of color).

Yasar is steadfast in his belief that leading LGBTQ advocacy organizations, like the Human Rights Campaign, define the success of the community by standards like marriage equality but fail to address the interests and needs of QTPOC. Despite this more layered understanding of what it means to be gay, Yasar's formation of gay identity is informed by search for freedom and connectedness with others, very much in sync with the men of the older generations. And like all gay men, he felt a connection with other boys at a young age, but he could not fully understand what this meant at the time okay:

> So I knew I liked boys when I was really, really young. I think I was like three. I just knew I liked this one little boy; it was actually when I was in Ghana and I knew I liked this one little boy. I just liked being around him. Yeah, just like playing with him.

Jeremy

At age 24, Jeremy is the only man of the Queer Generation interviewed to identify as HIV-positive. Jeremy speaks eloquently about being raised Catholic in a Dominican household, having sex with women during adolescence, and his conviction that he acquired HIV at a bathhouse. He is the first member of his family to partake in higher education, which he finds both an honor and a burden, a common experience for any first-generation scholar. Jeremy's life story has also been strongly shaped by growing up with an emotionally abusive father, an abuse that has persisted in the form of intimate partner violence, which is highly associated with substance use and sex risk.[10,11]

Much of Jeremy's narrative was sexually charged, as he strongly links sex with his identity as a gay man:

> To be a gay man, well, I'm interested, obviously, sexually and intimately to be with other men. So as a gay man, that's what I think of for me being a gay man.

Though Jeremy would often elaborate by adding ideas that were less rooted in sex, his first response to questions about his identity typically revolved around the act.

Common for many HIV-positive individuals, Jeremy came out as gay and HIV-positive at the same time, just like Emilio of the AIDS Generation. For these men, disclosure of sexual identity and HIV status becomes embedded in their life stories, causing the two identities to be highly associated with one another. Of course Jeremy realized he was gay long before he became HIV-positive and was aware of his same-sex attractions at a young age. Like many gay men of earlier generations, Jeremy dated women in high school, and his hypersexuality enabled him to have sex with them, but his attraction to men was clear to him. Still, he suppressed his sexual identity due to the perceived intolerance of his culture:

> When I first noticed that I liked men, I think that I was probably, like 11, 10, 11, around there. But I would always be in heavy denial because my parents are Dominican. They're from the Dominican Republic, and—I was the first generation to go to school. And so, yeah, it's not something that was acceptable, to be gay. . . . Like, I've met many people there—and I travel there a lot—who are out, and people are okay with that. But it's also something that a lot of people hide. A lot of men hide over there because it's not okay, or, like, traditionally, it's not okay. So I always hid it from myself, and I was in heavy denial through, I'd say, all of junior high school, high school. And I was dating girls. I was having sex with girls, but I knew that I did like men. So I started experimenting with men probably when I was 17.

Juan

Incredibly striking in his appearance, Juan, a 19-year-old NYU student, is the product of Mexican and Chinese parents. Though born in Mexico, he has traveled around the world with his family, living in Texas and Spain before settling in California. For Juan, like Yasar, religion has played a critical role in his life; he feared that his same-sex desires would land him in Hell, a lesson from his Catholic upbringing. So just like Jeremy, Emilio, and many other gay men learning about themselves, Juan dated a woman while growing up. He would convince her to go to gay clubs with him, and then he would sneak away to dark, back rooms.

Of course, even before then, he had an undeniable feeling that he would only later recognize as an attraction to men:

> I guess I always felt that way. I knew there was like something fundamentally different. And I used to play Barbies with my sister and I always wanted to be like Ken—or no, sorry—Barbie, so I could be with Ken.

When he turned 18, Juan actively came out to his family and many of his friends online via Facebook. In the short amount of time since, he has embraced this open identity in many ways, including a pink triangle tattoo as a vehicle to announce who he is and as a vehicle to come out in certain circumstances. As he says, "I'm owning this identity." The pink triangle is a notorious Nazi emblem that gay people were forced to wear in Germany in the '30s and '40s, later co-opted as a source of power by ACT UP, an international activist group, with social justice roots, that brought attention to AIDS in the 1980s—while the US government failed to attend to the disease—and challenged systems by which pharmaceutical treatments of HIV infection were tested and developed. This approach is reflected in the biohazard symbol many HIV-positive men sport today as a means of disclosing their status.

At this point in his emerging adulthood, Juan's identity as a gay man continues to be formed and will likely grow deeper as he ages. At the time of the interview, Juan was somber in his understanding of what it means to be a gay man:

> I think of someone who is part of a community, but also, at the same time, is going to constantly carry a stigma with them throughout their lives—well, like throughout my life.

Seeking to further clarify the burden that we as gay men experience, Juan succinctly and powerfully described the coming out process through which we all live—that seeming endless and lifelong reality:

> Like it's not something that people assume about you, or it's not—like society is not built to accommodate necessarily gay. It's a burden in that you have to like always clarify, always specify. You never know what people—your friends or like new people you meet are going to think.

FINAL THOUGHTS

Gay men of all generations have been forced to live with a fear of rejection by those whom we meet, by our families, by our religious communities. What heterosexual people fail to understand is that this fear of rejection permeates much of our lives, even excluding us from seemingly mundane experiences, like family holidays or other social events. To this day I relive a telephone call that I received from my aunt in the mid-1980s when she invited me to my cousin's college graduation party, making it abundantly clear that while I was invited, I was not welcome to bring a "friend."

It's possible to think about the experiences of gay men across the Stonewall, AIDS, and Queer generations in terms of a large great room in a home built in the early 1950s. Envision this room as a symmetrical square having windows on three walls. Across generations, the window treatments change from the blackout curtains, always drawn, of the Stonewall Generation; to the mini blinds of the AIDS Generation, letting in light, but which can quickly and discretely be closed; to the untreated window of the Queer Generation, allowing light to flood the room at all times. While these window treatments may shed light in different ways on the lives of the gay men in the room, what occurs in the room—in the heart and minds of gay men—is very much the same regardless of social visibility.

Perhaps the light creates for a more luminescent and liberating illusion inside the room, but the ones in the room are still negotiating what it means to be gay and how to be gay, finding and developing their identities, and deciding when, how, or if to come out to friends and family. These processes are consistent across time, but generational factors play a role, as is shown in comparing these men's stories of gay identification and disclosure. Integral to these generational differences are the specific crises each generation faces as well, the prominent societal or cultural struggles of the time that shape their world and become inseparable from the coming out process.

REFERENCES

1. Chan G, Bennett A, Buskin S, Dombrowski J, Golden M. Dramatic declines in lifetime HIV risk and persistence of racial disparities among men who have sex with men in King County, Washington, USA. Paper presented at International AIDS Society 2015; Vancouver, Canada.
2. Mimiaga MJ, Noonan E, Donnell D, et al. Childhood sexual abuse is highly associated with HIV risk-taking behavior and infection among MSM in the EXPLORE study. *J Acquir Immune Defic Syndr.* 2009;51(3):340–348.
3. Themstrom S, Orlov A, Handlin O. *Harvard encyclopedia of American ethnic groups.* Cambridge, MA: Belknap; 1980.

4. Burt S. The iceman cometh. *New York Times* 2018.

5. Taylor P, Keeter S. Millennials: confident. Connected. Open to Change. *Pew Research Center* 2010.

6. Carroll L, Gilroy PJ, Ryan J. Counseling transgendered, transsexual, and gender-variant clients. *J Couns Dev.* 2002;80(2):131–139.

7. The Kinsey Scale. 2018. https://kinseyinstitute.org/research/publications/kinsey-scale. php. Accessed July 6, 2018.

8. James SD. Gay man says Millennial term "Queer" is like the "N" word. *ABC News* 2013.

9. Eliason MJ. Identity formation for lesbian, bisexual, and gay persons: beyond a "minoritizing" view. *J Homosex.* 1996;30(3):31–58.

10. Stults CB, Javdani S, Greenbaum CA, Barton SC, Kapadia F, Halkitis PN. Intimate partner violence perpetration and victimization among YMSM: the P18 cohort study. *Psychol Sex Orientat Gend Divers.* 2015;2(2):152–158.

11. Stults CB, Javdani S, Greenbaum CA, Kapadia F, Halkitis PN. Intimate partner violence and substance use risk among young men who have sex with men: the P18 cohort study. *Drug Alcohol Depend.* 2015;154:54–62.

CHAPTER 2
Generational Crises

Much of today's fiction depicting gay life captures the beauty and consistency of lesbian, gay, bisexual, transgender, and queer (LGBTQ) struggles. The emotional conditions that color the storylines and characters of contemporary books, movies, plays, and TV shows about gay men are nuanced and complex, together creating a near renaissance of gay literature and entertainment. Consider George Falcone, the professor who loses his partner in Christopher Isherwood's 1964 novel *A Single Man*; or Jacob in Rabih Alameddine's *The Angel of History*, a coming-of-age story about a Yemeni-born man in San Francisco at the height of AIDS; or Craig and Hardy in David Levithan's young adult novel *Two Boys Kissing*. The latter is particularly powerful, as these young members of the Queer Generation go about their lives seeking to establish a record for world's longest kiss while the AIDS Generation echoes in the background, providing them with hope and support.

The impact of *Two Boys Kissing* also stems from the writer's relationship with his late uncle Robert "Bobby" Levithan, to whom that book is dedicated, who passed away in 2017 due to complications from AIDS. I knew Bobby as well. He was my colleague, friend, and an AIDS warrior who worked tirelessly to support those affected by, and infected with, HIV. I think of Bobby often, as so many men from the AIDS Generation think every day of their friends, partners, brothers, and family who were taken from them. But it's not just my generation that experiences this great loss— it has resonated throughout the years. While the AIDS Generation, and also the Stonewall Generation had nowhere to turn for guidance and support due to social climate exacerbated in part by the devastation of AIDS, neither did the Queer Generation. Miguel pointed out this challenge:

> *There's an entire generation of gay men who don't exist today because that [AIDS] wiped them out. And for that reason, I don't have any gay elders to look up to. So, like, it's just like, there's a whole generation of people that I could have, I could have had who don't exist today because of that.*

It could have been different for Miguel and his peers, and it may be for those who follow, in part due to the depiction of dynamic LGBTQ characters in mainstream entertainment. To the winds of change, Stephanos says of a gay-teen-centered sitcom, "TV just changed, I watched like *The Real O'Neals*, and it's like almost like alien to me that there would be such a thing." Emilio extended this idea, showing how much more than just TV has evolved, stating, "I can get married. I have equal protection under the law. I'm an equal citizen." Indeed these are advances.

Still, Emilio knows how much work remains:

> *I don't think two men can hold hands in every neighborhood across this nation. I just don't think it's safe to do that. That's the same through all generations.*

Every generation of gay men confronts its own crisis, though it is always based on one condition that cuts across time for all gay men: fear. The undeniable fear, precipitated by the crisis of each era, that no matter the strides we make, there is no future without challenges for gay men. The circumstances that shape the lives of each generation dictate the fear that exists within each cohort.

In his 2016 article[1] for Medium.com, "Fuck You, I'm Not a Millennial," author Patrick Hipp discusses how specific events or demarcation points that bring on sweeping change define generations, while the interval of years associated with each generation is less important. For the Stonewall Generation, the Stonewall Riots of 1969 began the liberation of gay identity; for the AIDS Generation, 1981 was the year in which the viral enemy was first encountered; and for the Queer Generation, the collapse of Lehman Brothers in 2008 set the wheels in motion that would define the economy for years to come, creating little room for financial success for many, and accompanied by ample opportunity for failure.

These challenges are palpable for the men coming of age and living through each crisis, but for those who preceded them, current challenges may seem obscure or minimal to what they had confronted. I've seen this mindset firsthand with members of the AIDS Generation who cannot bear witness to the difficulty of being a gay man in the 21st century, dismissing the behavior of younger men and diminishing their hardships, especially in relation to coming out. So, too, it is difficult for those in this moment to imagine the challenges of those who came before them. This inability to understand and communicate fully across the generations isn't a new concept, as intergenerational tensions in the gay community, and in general, have long existed.

Yet within the population of gay men, the need to break down these barriers and learn from each other is much more important, as we represent a small minority in a heterosexist society, a significant portion of which would prefer to ignore and silence us. Our power is in our numbers and in our ability to reach across the divide of the generations to create a collective voice. However, this unity can only begin by understanding what each generation faced, or currently faces, and by respecting the conditions that shape our formative years.

For example, a new generation of gay men today continues to fear HIV, but it is not their primary concern as it was for the generation that preceded them, nor should it be. Many members of the AIDS Generation, however, remain stuck in the year 1987 and believe the LGBTQ community must react to AIDS in the same way as it did then, failing to recognize that a new generation of gay men confronts a multitude of other challenges that we did not. Quite frankly, in light of advances in treatment, these new hurdles are potentially as debilitating as, though different from, the challenges created by AIDS.

Lorenzo, who came of age in the 1980s, summarizes how each generation faces its own crisis:

> I kinda was happy I came out when I did. I think it wasn't so, so bad. I mean, people becoming more acclimated to the idea. I really feel horrible for the generations before me, where they had nowhere to go. There was nobody out, per se. At that point, when I came out, there were people who had come out publicly and kinda had, you know, made those first ripples in the pond. And so, it wasn't such a foreign idea. But those poor men who couldn't come out and had to stay, you know, quiet, and live a life that was not meant to be lived, to me, like—you see, now, I'm getting emotional about it. In the latter generation, I think it became so easy to be gay. I'm not saying it's easy, but it was coming out—the coming out process was easy. It's never easy being gay. It really isn't. I mean, there's so much that goes with it. It's you coming out.

What's essential to realize is that these crises are cumulative: gay men of the Queer Generation struggle with the primary challenge of their time but still confront the challenges faced by the gay men of the preceding generations, namely acceptance and inclusion within society and the continued battle with AIDS. These problems may be somewhat ameliorated given the changing social landscape of the United States, and the biomedical advances in confronting AIDS, but they are still ever present. They are also further compounded by the challenges created by economic crisis.

In the end, each generation experiences the fear of coming out informed, in part, by the other life fears infusing that moment in time. These crises are shaped by the interplay of the social, cultural, political, legal, medical, and economic factors that create each period. It is within these contexts that the coming out experience must be understood, as coming out is both informed and precipitated by the crisis of each specific generation.

THE CRISIS OF IDENTITY

In the 1967 CBS documentary *The Homosexuals*, Mike Wallace reported, "The average homosexual—if there be such—is promiscuous. He is not interested in, nor capable of, a lasting relationship like a heterosexual marriage." When this documentary aired, the five men of the Stonewall Generation interviewed for this book (Jason, Jim, Ryan, Tom, and Wilson) would have ranged from early adolescence to young adulthood, formative years for any individual. At this young age, they were already experiencing the existential crisis that defined their generation, centered around realizing, actualizing, and living their gay identities at a time when homosexuality was illegal and where the disclosure of being gay could damage a person for the rest of his life.

Worse yet were the possibilities of being imprisoned, victimized, or killed. Gay men in countries outside the United States contended with similar social conditions, such as the Criminal Law Amendment Act of 1885 in Great Britain, under which the mathematician, computer scientist, and unsung World War II hero Alan Turing was chemically castrated because of his homosexuality. Brutality toward openly gay men—or even "suspected" gay men—was commonplace. Wilson recalls experiencing and witnessing such violence:

These drag queens had a female friend who went around with them. And they went into this bar, and the cops came in and said alright, you fucking faggots, blah-blah-blah-blah-blah. And they slammed this woman up against the wall thinking she was a drag queen, and tried to make her strip, so you know, they could find out— and she sued the police department for a fortune. And from that day on—this was way before, uh, Stonewall, I'm thinking.

Because of these circumstances, gay culture developed in the dark of night when men could meet with each other freely, often in fringe environments, where mainstream society wouldn't dare go. Wilson, who went to his first gay bar in 1956, describes the scene:

> Like, there were certain spots where you had to go down the stairs, and it was dark, and there were drills. They would go—if we turned the lights off, it means the cops are coming, and don't dance. There were places where you would—you could dance, but you had to know that if the lights blinked or something, you—you know, take your drink and go to the bar and stand, or take your drink and stand away. Don't be seen, when the cops come, with each other.

In a similar vein, Tom expressed the great fear and anxiety that he experienced while homosexuality was still illegal, contrasting the conditions pre and post Stonewall:

> It was in 1969; I was what, 20? 19? You know, it was just the beginning of the birth of the gay revolution. It was a time of celebration. [But] before that, it was not that. Absolutely, it was not that. I remember, uh, when I came to New York, I had friends—two gay guys—who lived here, and I stayed with them, and I think we went out to a bar called Christopher's End, and it was still a time when we could have been rounded up, and I wasn't of an age that I guess I could—I wasn't even supposed to be there, I don't remember. I felt afraid. I was fearful, because I saw what had happened, historically, to gay people, but then I saw what was happening with the gay revolution. So, you know, there was fear over here, and there was hope over here, and, you know, the arrow of time goes only one direction. I thought, "Well, you know, eventually . . . "—but how quickly? Back then, we didn't know. My friend Felix, who's 87, I guess—87 years old. He was a dancer. He danced with Judy Garland's boys, and, yeah, I think he was arrested, along with one of his friends.

The identity crises for the men of Stonewall caused them to compartmentalize their personalities, creating multiple personas in order to survive. Such inauthenticity creates psychological tension and disconnection, preventing the integration of multiple identities into one whole, leaving the person feeling fractured and incomplete. Jim traces this crisis to an early age:

> Growing up in Queens [New York] in the '50s offered my parents no opportunity to think outside the norms that Ozzie and Harriet presented. Being gay was a mysterious/deadly curse and lumped into the box with the "C" word, cancer. "No one" was gay, at least in our immediate circle and even Liberace was thought of as a fun showman.

For gay men, particularly gay white men, efforts to pass as straight were common. Few were honest, open, and proud, especially before the Stonewall Riots. Such a suppression of feelings caused many men to avoid coming out, even if their sexual identity was difficult to hide.

Lorenzo, although a member of the AIDS Generation, attests to a similar reality when speaking about his father, who had owned a gay bar and whom Lorenzo believes was most likely gay himself:

> I think my dad did what he was supposed to do. I honestly believe he did what he felt he had to do, rather than what he wanted to do.

As a young man, Jim hid his identity for years until he decided to come out to his parents. He had envisioned an incredibly negative reaction from his family, and upon disclosing his sexual identity, they responded by sending him to a conversion therapist. As mentioned in chapter 1, Jim was later able to use his identity to avoid being sent to the Vietnam War. Jim shared the details of his recruitment day:

> They said, "What do you have?" And I said, "I have a letter." "Yeah. Okay." And very dismissive, and "All right, give us the letter." So you're walking what felt like you know, 50 feet, you know, in front of the world, fully dressed uniform people, fully naked guys back here, and, and I present the letter, and they open it up, and I'm back in line again. And they passed the letter among themselves. And the first thing they said was, "You suck dick." And the hush came over the room. It was like, "Oh, my God. I'm out." And you know. "Do you get fucked, too?" And so there, in these series of questions, and—I had to admit, "Yes." And you know, and of course, you're not speaking loud enough for them, so you had to shout in this big, what could've been a gym, "Yes. Yes. Yes." Much to their dismay, they had to give me you know, whatever they stamped, that I'm not fit for service. It was a big relief for me. But then I harbored the idea. [But] I put that aside. Nobody else knew; I kept it all a secret.

In the 2010 film *Beginners*, Christopher Plummer portrays an older gay man—a member of the Stonewall Generation—who finally comes out after a life of pretending to be straight when his wife passes away. Paralleling fiction, the documentary *On My Way Out: The Secret Life of Nani and Popi* depicts the life of Roman Blank, a 95-year-old Holocaust survivor who came out after 65 years of marriage to his wife. In the film, Blank states, "For 90 years I was in pain—and still am. I never let you know or feel what is going on in my heart. Never until now."[2]

These depictions of the Stonewall Generation's crisis are demonstrative of the challenges of coming out. For many gay men of this time, systematic oppression and social stigmatism left them with choices that were less than ideal: suppress their identities, never come out, and isolate themselves or only act on their sexual desires when they could sneak away for a few minutes from the ideal "All-American" families they had built. For a subset of other men who did not take one of those paths, the choice was to come out quietly and secretly only within a small circle, hiding a huge part of themselves from society at large and never fully integrating their identities nor living their true authentic lives.

Despite the despicable social conditions, this generation of gay Baby Boomers began evening the playing field for gay men, much as all Baby Boomers did for future generations, as noted by one of the original *Saturday Night Live* writers Marilyn Suzanne Miller:[3] "for political activism, for the right to wear insane clothes and crazily short skirts, for the right to get married outside and that fact that we are all saying give peace a chance." Their coming out, or lack thereof, was influenced and framed by the social circumstances that denounced being gay as both pathological and criminal. They had to battle criminalization, institutionalization, and societal norms, actively putting up fronts of resistance to make any progress forward. Unfortunately, these social epidemics would be ongoing for the generation that followed, exacerbated by a biological epidemic.

THE CRISIS OF AIDS

For a large portion of the AIDS Generation, coming out is not only tied to their sexual orientation but also to their HIV status, as seen with Emilio in the previous chapter. Concerns about rejection from family and friends are thus compounded—that fear of the unknown, of a precarious future or none at all. This sense of hopelessness is encapsulated in the words of one man after having watched an early AIDS film: "My future didn't look very promising based on the movie's depiction of what was to come."

This fear of coming out for HIV-positive men is perpetuated within the gay community itself through repeated disclosure of HIV status to sexual partners. While often met with respect and dignity, status disclosure by HIV-positive men is too often met with rejection and hostility, embodied in the use of the phrase "I am clean" to signal HIV-negative status. Though the Stonewall Generation opened the floodgates, promising a new sexual freedom for the generation to follow, HIV unraveled that promise.

Seth was astute in his description of the situation, showing how the need for connection among gay men in a homophobic world mingled with the growing HIV crisis, creating chaos in their lives:

> We had only just found our feet as a society, as a subculture. And it was this disease, this loss, HIV and/or AIDS, and this disease of unattainable intimacy, this constant search for intimacy, um, that would lead us more and more to this wanting to feel alive. . . . And just like, over and over again, exposing ourselves, exposing our immune systems to essentially being run down, you know, origins of HIV aside, the fact that we were damaging our immune systems to be so susceptible was a big piece. And I think it has everything to do with self-esteem, a need to break free from the bonds of self-loathing, um, that being next to impossible in that period.

AIDS began to define coming out. As awareness about the epidemic grew within the gay community, it complicated an already complex process of gay identity development. By the first half of the 1980s, being gay, coming out, and having sex with other men were all covered with an ominous cloud, as noted by Lorenzo:

> Well, don't forget the time—pardon me if I throw us into a group here—but it's because of our age bracket. The fear of god was put into us about this: you didn't touch anybody; you wouldn't do anything.

Moreover, the social conditions of the time segregating the "innocent victims of AIDS," namely hemophiliacs and children, from those who "brought the disease upon themselves," such as gay men and injection drug users, served to only further stigmatize gay men's lives. When asked about how AIDS defined his coming out as a gay man, Emilio bulleted a set of films and television programs that defined his formative years. Of *The Ryan White Story*, which aired on ABC in 1989, Emilio said:

> I recall seeing this film and it stirred up feelings of sadness. It was hard to hear about the story of this child with HIV. At that time he was considered an "innocent victim." When I heard this terminology it made me feel shame. Back then, I felt like I was a "guilty" victim since I contracted the virus sexually.

The AIDS crisis unfolded a mere decade after we had begun developing our rights. In effect this event defined the generation's formative years and would shape the members' lives for decades to come. The impact that the virus has had on gay men of the generation and their willingness to come out and live openly cannot be understated: AIDS affected their physical, emotional, and social well-being, the very core elements to which resilient seropositive gay men have fought gallantly to maintain while living with this chronic disease. The influence of the virus on all aspects of well-being comes from the fact that the HIV crisis in the United States is as much a viral as it is a social phenomenon.

This social aspect was especially apparent during the '80s and early '90s when openly discriminatory policies were created by the government and accepted by the public. Consider the censored prevention posters from the early days of AIDS, both provocative and erotic in nature, which celebrated gay sexuality and a sense of beauty while warning about the virus, forcing people to pay attention. The Helms Amendment struck down the use of these images in 1987, allowing for the persistence of more negative imagery. For Lorenzo, the first images of gay men that he recalls as he was coming of age were far from positive:

> The frail gaunt figures covered in lesions, men not in control of themselves and the sunken eyes. I buried these in the recesses of my mind quickly, not one really wants to face reality. I was kinda pissed. Here I was finally old enough to address the feelings I had and this disease, this unbeatable thing was there to stop me. I stuck my head in the sand, crossing my fingers that what I saw in those early depictions would never be me. I remember being in the clubs back then, anytime we saw someone who had lost a few pounds it was assumed that he was sick. I don't recall the term HIV Positive back then, just sick.

The deterioration of social networks followed. Men born between 1960 and 1964, the group of gay men in the United States with highest infection rates, would have been 18 between 1978 and 1982, a time of sexual awaking for many emerging adults. At that point in time, though, the virus was very much in the midst of the gay community and awareness was limited. The disease devastated this new generation's community, shaping their social and personal lives in the moment and for decades to follow. It's no surprise that the coming out experience of gay men of the AIDS Generation has been described as coming "Out of the Closet and into the Trenches."[4]

Despite these circumstances, we persevered, we fought back, and we demonstrated our resilience. Reviewing David France's book, How to Survive a Plague, the political commentator Andrew Sullivan, an HIV-positive gay man of the AIDS Generation, asked:[5]

> A question has always hung over the reaction of gay men to the plague that terrorized and decimated them in the 1980s and 1990s: Why did they not surrender? . . . Why, after a brief moment of liberation in the 1970s, did they not crawl back into the closet and die?

In 1994, Pedro Zamora, an HIV-positive gay man and AIDS activist, appeared on one of the first reality TV shows *The Real World* on MTV. Of Zamora, Emilio stated:

> I remember feeling empowered when Pedro was on "The Real Life." It was so awesome to see someone with the virus being so honest and open about who he was. It made me feel supported in my openness about my status.

A battle for tolerance was compounded with the proliferation of the viral pathogen, first derailing and then activating the gay civil rights movement of the AIDS Generation. AIDS provided a momentary setback by perpetuating the ignorance of many and justifying their intolerance of gay men. Alternatively the AIDS epidemic gave us a face, thrust us front and center, and required that we come out from the dark of night to face the light, albeit a gloomy one. Once we came out, we would never go back again.

THE CRISIS OF FAILURE

The crisis of today's Millennial generation comes from a worldview influenced by major political upheaval, identity politics, financial and economic instability, and the chaotic nature of a post-9/11 reality, leading to disillusionment and a sense of uncertainty. The financial crisis of 2008, in particular, created subpar and unfavorable life conditions, especially for gay men of color, providing fewer opportunities to develop one's place in the world. Such diminished economic conditions can directly affect how, and if, someone comes out. Yasar expressed this idea clearly:

> [How easy it is] to come out it depends like on your economic status. Like can you financially support yourself if worse comes to worst. Like if you were kicked out of your home could you support yourself? Or do you have a network of people that can help you. And location as well, if I were to come out in like Charlotte or like a smaller town versus in New York. There are more services, and if I were to kicked out and be homeless, there are more services in New York or here than in a smaller town. But coming to now, there are more services in general. Especially in New York and especially in bigger cities. But is it easier [than older generations]? Hmm I'm not exactly sure.

At its core, the financial crisis has left an indelible mark on the lives of many members of the Queer Generation. Jeremy, who was a teenager at the time of this great economic crash, described the situation as such:

The financial crisis of 2007 affected my family greatly. I remember my mother getting laid off and a cloud of devastation hovered over our house for quite sometime. Our dinners were becoming smaller for the time being since my father was the only one being able to provide while my mother looked for other jobs. I found myself looking for side jobs after school, but I wasn't of age. I can say that they weren't the best times financially, but our love for each other and sense of family kept us together and I remember all the weekly gatherings we had with our aunts, uncles, and cousins. We would all go to one household and make a big meal which all the adults would chip in for. My family made the best with what they had. . . . Later in 2008, my mother got approved for NYC Housing section 8, and that changed our lives a bit. We were able to move into somewhere bigger, and financially we were way more stable than that previous year.

According to the US Bureau of Labor,[6] during 2017–2018, unemployment rates for men between ages 20 and 24 hovered between 7% and 8%. For 25- to 34-year-old men, the rate was around 4% in this period. These figures are even more troubling for young men of color. Moreover, *Forbes Magazine* reports[7] that recent college graduates spend approximately $350 per month in student loan payments. In light of average starting salaries, this cost translates to an 8% to 10% reduction in salary for roughly a decade after these Millennials graduate.

Financial burdens are quite real for Miguel, who left home when he was around 16 after the harsh reaction he received from his family when he came out:

There was this, like, poverty looming over my head. I didn't have a job. I didn't have any money. I didn't have any, really, anywhere to go. So I had I had to drop out of high school. I had to get a job. Started working at this pretzel store thing at, like, Faneuil Hall.

Yasar also had to find a means to support himself, and pay his college tuition, when his parents refused to help him financially after he came out and then actively tried to break down his identity as a gay man:

I was like drinking a lot; I was drinking like basically every day. And I stayed up a lot 'cause I was also working three jobs junior year and I was like taking 19 credit hours.

To this day, both Miguel and Yasar struggle with their careers and finances. In fact, developing a career has been challenging for every young man of the Queer Generation with whom I spoke. Even Reid, whose parents are upper middle class, constantly grapples with his next career move, and in the interim, he bartends at an upscale restaurant in the East Village. When asked how his upbringing has influenced his life today, Reid described how his parents sheltered him and the impact that had:

> I honestly feel like being overprotected and graduating during the economic decline created failure. My parents, I think, tried to protect me and my sister from life (i.e.: I wasn't allowed to watch The Simpsons for being too inappropriate, never had the sex talk, not talking about budgeting but just making us work to get into the workforce). I feel like maybe I wasn't ready for life and what it had to offer, but I also came up when social media was rising, so it was nice to see that I wasn't the only one struggling. However, because my parents sheltered me, I feel I wasn't really aware of how much job opportunity, social, culture, etc. . . . opportunity there was out there, which was the biggest failure. Until I moved out of my parent's house, my entire view on life was blinded by what my parents had given me.

It could be argued that these conditions and struggles are simply the circumstances that all young people face as they develop their careers. But I disagree. Today, even with a graduate degree, many young people go unemployed or underemployed. With the current economic conditions, younger Americans are turning their backs on higher education. The hope and promise for an illustrious career held by a college degree have all but vanished. These conditions make it difficult to take positive risks in one's career, and they increase the costs of failure.

Jeremy summarized the problem, tying together the economy with his social class, culture, and upbringing:

> Throughout my life, economic conditions in the US affected my family greatly. A lot of it was because my parents had no more than a high school diploma and didn't have the opportunity to better their education due to choosing to come to the US to give my siblings and I a better life. There was very little space for failure since they pressured us to excel in our studies because they knew how important it was for us to get a good education and have good careers in the future. My peers in the Latin community dealt with very similar ways of parenting from their parents. It's as if we were all being disciplined the same way. Our role models, or adults in our lives, left no room for risk or choice of not going to college. When I was 18 years old, if I was to tell my parents I wanted to take a year off of school and pitch an idea for a new business, they would look at me like I've lost my mind.

Such circumstances may be even more insurmountable, and financial realities even worse, for gay and gender nonconforming individuals of color, as Yasar describes:

> *I mean yeah, I can marry somebody like another man, but again my trans sisters are being killed and they're being homeless and they're getting into sex work. Which is a valid source of income, it's a valid job. But I mean, sometimes most of the times that's their only source of income and then cause they're not receiving the proper jobs that they need to survive.*

These financial realities for the men of the Queer Generation are best exemplified in Miguel's life experience. Having managed to survive after coming out and leaving his parents' home for two years, Miguel returned to seek their help to pursue an education:

> *I showed up. She was there. She gave me a hug. We sat down and talked in the kitchen, and I let her know everything that had happened in, like, the subsequent, like, two years that I was gone. She hadn't really heard from me or even knew if I was alive or dead, you know, so just kind of trying to reassure her that I was very much alive and that I was just doing fine without her. And but there was an issue. It was that I wanted to go to school. I couldn't go to school without them helping me. So she was just, like, all right, let's sign these papers. Let's put this in motion. She's like, I do want to see you go to college. So I apply to school. I get in.*

After receiving his bachelor's degree, Miguel hoped to achieve his pharmacy doctorate, but he was unable to support this next step in his education, leading to his current circumstances:

> *So I graduated with a bachelor's and I haven't been able to do anything with it since. My parents, like, my dad specifically signed one of loans—mind you we [my dad and I] still haven't really talked [since I came out]. I'm in a fuck ton of debt. I'm trying to find a job that's higher than a pharmacy technician program. I can't find anything. And I am stuck. I have a fuck ton of debt. I have nowhere to [live], I actually had to end up moving back in with my parents for that summer because I had no job. I have a degree that's basically useless. So I have a useless degree. I am now 24, 25 years old, having gone and done a four-year program, really regretting having done it. I am now back at my parent's place, like, living in my own bedroom for that summer, and, uh, my father's not talking to me. My mother is, is on board, but she just is kind of disappointed that I haven't been the wild success that I was supposed to be.*

Miguel's story is a compelling encapsulation of the ongoing challenges for the men of the Queer Generation. As writer and anthropologist Sarah Kendzior points out, having lived the majority of their adult lives in the shadow of the Great Recession, they "have lower incomes, less mobility, and greater financial dependence on older relatives than any other generation in modern history." She goes on to state, "many Millennials do not have a lot of choice. They are merely reacting to lost opportunity."[8] And like most Americans few if any will be in the top 1% of the country that holds the majority of the wealth.

Coming out for the Queer Generation may not be fraught with the illegality of homosexuality faced by the members of the Stonewall Generation, nor of the uncertainty of surviving AIDS, but the process presents its own challenges. Millennials have inherited the previous generations' economic failures and the ensuing fallout. Twenty years from now the aftermath of the recession will likely still be felt. These conditions result in a crisis of failure for the gay men of the Queer Generation as they try to fight to make their ways in the world, affecting how, when, or if they come out. Some members of previous generations demean this experience, but it must be seen as simply a new and different struggle than those who preceded them faced, making it no better or worse, and also as a continuation of the overall struggle gay men have dealt with for the past 50 years. That said, it's not always easy to convince these generations to see eye to eye on the importance of the crises they experience.

INTERGENERATIONAL DYNAMICS

Generations bleed into each other. They exist on a continuum that transitions from one generation to the next with commonalities and a period of overlap. As mentioned in the beginning of the chapter, the crises of each generation are therefore cumulative. I have little patience for those of my generation, or of the Stonewall Generation, who consider the Queer Generation as privileged, entitled, lazy, and unable to understand earlier struggles, especially in regards to AIDS. Unfortunately, I have spoken to many men who take this point of view, and I think they do so to their detriment as they fail to understand today's crisis for the Queer Generation. In many ways, it comes down to a lack of communication.

Encouraging communication across generations is not an easy feat and it plays out in how members of an older set point fingers at those "young crazy kids." Many men of the AIDS Generation who have been living with HIV throughout their lives suggest that younger men do not fear AIDS enough, disregard its severity, and don't respect the circumstances through which members of the AIDS Generation lived. It has been found that while HIV and other health issues burden the Queer Generation, the other problems discussed earlier in this chapter, nested within the economic and social conditions of their own time, are prevalent.[9]

To connect better across these generations, and work together, it's important to understand the crises of each other's specific cohort. However, when leaders like author and gay rights advocate Larry Kramer chide and berate younger gay men, as he did in a November 7, 2004, speech at Cooper Union in New York City, it's obvious there has been a breakdown in communication and the opening of a divide:

> *Most gay people I see appear to act as if they're bored to death. Too much time in your hands, my mother would say. Hell, if you have time to get hooked on crystal and do your endless sex-seeking, you have too much time on your hands. Ah, you say you want to have a little fun? "Can't I get stoned and try barebacking at least one time?" ARE YOU OUT OF YOUR FUCKING MIND! At this moment in our history, no, you cannot. Anyway, we had your fun and look what it got us into. And it is still getting us into. You kids want to die? Because that's what I sometimes think. Well, then die.*[10]

How such a tirade would help anybody of any generation is unclear. Instead, these words contribute to an even greater chasm between generations.

For many of my peers Larry Kramer is a hero. During the height of AIDS he founded ACT UP and cofounded the first AIDS service organization, Gay Men's Health Crisis (GHMC). His efforts are monumental elements of gay history in the fight for our rights, health, and safety. But, speeches like the one at Cooper Union demonstrate the worldview of a man unable to see anything outside himself and an inability to show any sense of empathy, even though he recognizes that part of what these young men want is what he has already had (i.e., "Anyway, we had your fun and look what it got us into."). Perhaps there was a better way to deliver this message. Importantly, this type of attitude demonstrates how we as an older generation of gay men are very much at fault in perpetuating this ongoing intergenerational dynamic.

The inability of gay men to speak with each other across generations is a missed opportunity, as they fail to take full advantage of each other's knowledge and experience to learn from one another. It is oversimplistic to believe that younger men simply dismiss older men and the crises they have had to manage, a popular opinion among the AIDS Generation. The older generations are as responsible for this ineffective crosstalk as their younger peers, although if we have a very clear lesson from the 2016 Philadelphia Pride March at which a new more inclusive LGBTQ flag was revealed, it is that a new generation has a voice and power that must be heard and respected. New and developing ideas, terms, and lifestyles within the

LGBTQ community sometimes leave older generation members confused or skeptical. One such concept is gender fluidity, of which Ryan, a member of the Stonewall Generation, said:

> What the Hell is pansexual? Is this when you have sex in a frying pan or you tell someone you want 12 inches and you want it to hurt so you fuck them 3 times and hit them in the head with a frying pan?

Though humorous, Ryan's sentiments are found throughout his generation and they directly affect the relationship between these generations. For Millennials, gay or straight, gender fluidity or pansexuality—attraction to a variety of gender and sexual identities, in which gender roles, gender identity, and sexual preference are less defined and more open—are becoming mainstream, while older people, also gay or straight, are sometimes left scratching their heads, having been socialized in a society of binaries. In such a climate, it can be difficult for some to accept these new realities and work to understand the issues affecting today's LGBTQ community. It's no wonder some gay men believe that coming of age today is a joyride compared to the past—if they haven't taken the time to listen, and instead prioritize vocalizing their own judgments, then they'll be blinded to what's happening, rooting themselves in a false sense of reality.

However, there is a ray of hope. Groups like the Generations Project are building intergenerational dialogue through storytelling and other events. Despite his joking comments about pansexuality, Ryan has been a leader in sharing his life experiences with younger men, who are highly receptive to hearing his life story:

> Earlier this summer, in honor of this woman Jane who—saved Washington Square Park—the one who fought Robert Moses—they had all these walking tours and they had it on Facebook. And one walking tour was walking to all the old gay infamous clubs. And of course, one of those was the Anvil, another one was Crisco Disco, another one was the Mine Shaft. And so I sent a note—I says, you boys—these boys were 20 something years old, you know? Children. So, I sent a little note. I said, I'd love to do a tour with you—boys will know—you won't know who I am, but I was the—I was the star of the Anvil. I'd love to do it, if you want me to talk or anything. I'd be happy to. If not, I'd just love to come. Get a note back, we know who you are. Hi, we would love for you to come and please feel free to talk. So, I go and I'm thinking, oh it's gonna be these two boys and ten old queens like me reminiscing about the past. There were like 70 people there. They wanted to know the history.

In a similar vein, Seth believes that this dynamic across the generations is improving. He sees older gay men as providing hope and optimism through a blissful, yet supportive voyeurism, watching a new set of young men emerge into their lives as gay:

> I suppose men look to boys as the next generation. So it's their responsibility to train them. But I think there's also a sense of connection to their own youthfulness, a connection to their own sense of worth, that we, you know, stay alive because of our relationship to younger men and what it means to be alive in society through the eyes of someone who is just approaching it from that standpoint. This, you know, this beginner's mind. Just finding, you know, something that we can begin to relate to on our own level.

Ultimately the responsibility of gay men as elder statesmen should be akin to the supportive voice of the AIDS Generation that resonates throughout *Two Boys Kissing*—to leave things better for those who follow and to hope that conditions continuously improve. The success of these efforts cannot rest on their shoulders alone, nor should hubris prevail on them to think they can manage this on their own. Instead, with the development of intergenerational dynamics and intergenerational dialogue, attempts to improve the lives of all gay men will be best realized, and together we can combat the crises of today, the wounds of the past, and the inevitable crises of tomorrow.

FINAL THOUGHTS

Each generation faces unique struggles onset by the social, cultural, political, and economic environments of the time, but the coming out struggle is universal and one of the most powerful phenomena that ties all gay men. Gay men across generations experience a fear that there will be no future or that the future is riddled with little possibility, affecting how, when, or if they decide to disclose their sexual identity. The crises of the three generations—identity, AIDS, and failure—build on one another, painting a portrait of the gay experience that can be scary or disheartening, especially for those of us who live it. Only through understanding between generations can we ensure a sense of hope and survival.

Even with an increased and more dynamic portrayal of LGBTQ characters in mainstream entertainment and elsewhere, advances in the battle against AIDS, and a decrease in the government's limitations over our lives—though they still exist in parts of the country—coming out has not necessarily become easier for the Queer Generation. Like the gayborhoods in New York City that made their way from the Christopher Street area of the Stonewall era, to Chelsea of the AIDS era, to Midtown and the East Village of the early Queer era, the men who navigated these neighborhoods at those respective times were on the fringe—and in many ways we've stayed there. Without each other's support, we will continue to be marginalized, and the lifelong process of coming out may never become easier.

REFERENCES

1. Hipp P. Fuck you, I'm not a Millennial. *Medium* 2016.
2. Bielski Z. The joy and pain of LGBTQ seniors living openly for the first time. *Globe and Mail* 2017.
3. Miller MS. Why are the Baby Boomers in such a bad mood? *New York Times* 2017.
4. Rosenfeld D, Bartlam B, Smith RD. Out of the closet and into the trenches: gay male Baby Boomers, aging, and HIV/AIDS. *Gerontologist.* 2012;52(2):255–264.
5. Sullivan A. The AIDS fight: Andrew Sullivan on a history of the movement. *New York Times* 2016.
6. Bureau of Labor Statistics. Labor force statistics from the current population survey. 2018. https://www.bls.gov/web/empsit/cpseea10.htm. Accessed July 8, 2018.
7. Landrum S. The impact of student loan debt on Millennial happiness. *Forbes* 2017.
8. Kendzior S. The myth of millennial entitlement was created to hide their parents' mistakes. *Quartz* 2016.
9. Halkitis PN, Cook SH, Ristuccia A, et al. Psychometric analysis of the Life Worries Scale for a new generation of sexual minority men: the P18 Cohort Study. *Health Psychol.* 2018;37(1):89–101.
10. Kramer L. *The tragedy of today's gays.* New York, NY: Tarcher; 2005.

CHAPTER 3
Being

In 2010 *The Guardian* reported[1] the findings of a poll conducted by Stonewall, a community-based organization in the United Kingdom seeking to empower the lesbian, gay, bisexual, transgender, and queer (LGBTQ) population locally and globally, in which they asked 1,500 openly LGBTQ people about the age at which they had come out. Among older adults, age 60 and above, the average age when they had come out was 37; for those in their 30s the average was 21; and among those 18 to 24, it was 17. Though this survey was taken in the United Kingdom and there is wide geographic variation, especially considering less tolerant and more homophobic nations, these ages align with those of gay men in the United States. The trend is obvious—with each generation gay men have started coming out at a younger age.

Representative of this change, you need look no further than gay men in pop music. In 2016, the documentary *Freedom* about George Michael's life and music was released, not long before Sam Smith's record *The Thrill of It All*. In the meantime, Elton John had been preparing for his "Farewell Yellow Brick Road" Tour, claimed to be his last, in which he plans to play more than 300 shows around the world from the fall of 2018 through 2021. It is serendipitous that such milestones in these three men's careers were crossing over as I was writing this book. *Freedom* ended up in repeat mode on my DVR; *The Thrill of It All* became background music for me as I compiled these interviews; and I rediscovered Elton John's classic 1973 record *Goodbye Yellow Brick Road* (dare I show my generational biases, the album was on vinyl when I first bought it the year it was released—ergo for me, it will always be a "record" not a "compact disc" or "digital download").

Elton John, George Michael, and Sam Smith are emblematic of the three generations of gay men from the '50s through today. Though they are all British white cisgender males, their lives are symbolic of many of the themes that emerge both within and across the generations and quite powerfully demonstrate the struggles of coming out. Most of Elton John's early life was spent "in the closet," ridden with alcohol and substance abuse, even marrying Renate Blaeul, a female German recording engineer, in the 1980s. Like so many men of the AIDS generation, George Michael's life was defined in great part by the loss of a partner, Anselmo Feleppa, to complications of AIDS in 1993. This trauma affected him for many years, as articulated on his masterful recording *Older* released in 1996. Michael still didn't "officially" come out in public, however, until 1998 during an interview with CNN.[2]

Smith's experience was different from both John's and Michael's, publicly embracing his identity early on, along with a fluidity in gender and the intersection of his sexuality and gender, as noted in an interview he gave to *The Sunday Times*[3] during the release of *The Thrill of It All*: "I don't know what the title would be, but I feel just as much woman as I am man." Despite the fact that Smith is a Millennial coming of age at a time when Western society is somewhat more embracing of LGBTQ people than in the past, he nonetheless expressed the stress of realizing his sexual identity: "Coming out is really difficult. Even if you're in the most amazing situation with the most understanding parents, which I was lucky enough to have, it is so difficult coming out. Just saying the words out loud and having to do it is actually ridiculous and intense."

Both Elton John and George Michael didn't have the benefits of a more open society, as they came of age and strove for success in a homophobic world, but their experiences are illustrative of the continuous aspect of coming out. Before his marriage Elton John had publicly stated that he believed all people were somewhat bisexual, and George Michael had come out to some of his family members—though not his parents—earlier in life. Even with Sam Smith performing as an openly gay person, he too had to deal with the difficulties—the ridiculousness and intensity—of coming out and essentially still has to, every time he's interviewed on the subject.

Today, the expression "coming out of the closet" has become antiquated, as the *Queerty* staff writers pointed out in a 2010 piece, "Can We Please Come Up With a New Way to Say 'Coming Out'?"[4] While the term "coming out" is used throughout this book, it is a mere representation of the experience. Just as the title of this chapter implies, the state of being true to one's self can be swapped for "coming out"—a continuous act that LGBTQ people must contend with every day, a part of their existence in a heteronormative society. Unlike our heterosexual peers who benefit from being raised in such a society, we confront the perpetual need to explain and clarify who we are. I challenge any straight person to try explaining that they are straight at work or in school, or to a family member, knowing full well that this disclosure will be met with a level of confusion, concern, and anger typically saved for gay identity disclosure—trust us, it's not easy. (The film *Love, Simon* deftly depicts this idea, but I said it first.) As sexual minority individuals we spend our lives coming out, a burden most cannot even fathom. It is an ongoing process that lasts a lifetime—in perpetuity, perhaps—that people like Thomas even in his 60s, continues to grapple with:

> *Coming out is a lifelong experience. Every time I experience internal homophobia, I realize that's a place where I haven't come out yet, where I feel uncomfortable just being who I am. You know, I haven't truly become comfortable with me as a person, the authentic me, and here, at almost 67 years old, I think, "What the fuck?" You know, um, but it still happens.*

REALIZING AND RECONCILING

For many years "homosexuality" was seen as either a disease that must be treated or a phase that a young person would outgrow en route to a "normal" heterosexual adult life. This false narrative and misunderstanding has dominated history in the era of the Abrahamic religions, namely Judaism, Christianity, and Islam, and persists in some places today. Such misconceptions provide fodder to reparative therapeutic approaches seeking to "cure" people of being gay, a type of therapy that has been outlawed in many jurisdictions, locally and globally, but continues to have the backing of some like Jack Nicolosi, a clinical psychologist who, up to his death in March 2017, argued in favor of such treatments.[5]

It's disheartening that this disease-based view of homosexuality persists while continuing to fuel religious zealots. Growing up in the Greek Orthodox Church, I was aware of this factually incorrect view that the church espoused on a whole, but the recent words of Eleftherios Tatsis, an Australian Greek Orthodox priest, cut to the bone nonetheless, when in 2017 he suggested that those in his congregation who voted in favor of same-sex marriage in Australia should be shot; he later apologized.[6]

This level of intolerance creates long-term psychological damage for young people who are still processing their identity and who are most vulnerable during their childhood. As noted in the words of Yasar:

> *Oh my gosh, so I remember when I was young I was really scared I was going to hell. So like every night I would sleep with my, I shared a room with my middle brother, and um like after he would go to sleep um, I would like pray for like 30*

minutes. I would be like crying and stuff and like, "Yo I don't want to go to hell." And I remember this one time when we started going to the small White southern Baptist church. We got baptized, so it like washed our sins away. I was like, "Yo I'm so happy" because I'm saying I'm like not gonna be gay, I'm not gonna have any gay thoughts like it's gonna be great. But then like, by the end of the week I was like yeah, that's not happening, so I was constantly trying to like pray it away and it just never worked.

Such circumstances tend to postpone or stop people from coming out, in turn delaying their own self-understanding or denying their personal development, their ability to simply be.

As we come into our own as gay men, we must go through three stages of development: interpretation, internalization, and reconciliation.[7] By learning who we are, incorporating into our selves, and integrating it into our overall being, we can achieve and maintain our gay identity. In this process, we transition from childhood, with no sense of ourselves aside from whatever directly surrounds us, to adolescence, in which we develop an understanding that we are separate from our social and physical environments, to adulthood, the universalistic stage in which we realize that we can evaluate social norms.[8] Only until an individual can be mindful and critical of such norms can gay identity be fully realized, a process that may occur over decades, shaped by the mores of the time.

Coming of age in a more enlightened era, this evaluative process and full integration of gay identity for members of the Queer Generation could possibly be abbreviated and potentially less burdensome. However there is no guarantee, especially given the social circumstances that shape the diverse cultures in the United States, as seen in Miguel's experiences growing up in Chelsea, Massachusetts, right outside Boston:

When my mom got pregnant with me, they [my parents] just, kind of, decided to settle in Massachusetts outside of Boston. I grew up in a very, like, interesting multicultural community. There were a lot of—anyone who had been in the war, like, with the United States at any point in time had some kind of community there. So there was like a Vietnamese community from the '70s that still existed there. There was, um, there was still remnants of, like, Jewish people who were still there from, like, you know, like, when they were immigrating to the U.S. from, like, World War II . . . the small Korean population. There was an Afghani population. There was a Bosnian population, um, literally, any, like, up until recent period. There were lots of different kids speaking lots of different languages. So I grew up with the idea— the notion of this America that it was very multicultural. I got, um—growing up though, like, with each and every one of those cultures—though none of them were ever really accepting of gay people though. Like just the way that people would talk. Like, there was—whether, whether they were, like, saying "faggot" to you in

English or "pato" in, like, Puerto Rican, or, like, like, or—I forget what the Bosnian term for it was—but they didn't like you. Like, you stood out. Straightness was— or, like, hetero-normity was, is norm, the norm, the thing that connected everybody together.

Nineteen-year-old Juan had a similar experience growing up in a multicultural family, with a Mexican father and Chinese mother:

My dad, every time he saw like a gay couple. He'd be like, "Oh, maricon," and were like look away and stuff like that. I think it was like—subconsciously I was just like burying that deeper and deeper. Like every time I saw that, oh this is really not okay. Or like, oh this is absolutely not acceptable. And obviously, I would play along with my dad and be like, "Oh, yeah, that's gross."

In addition to these cultural concerns, there are political and social ones as well. With recent political conditions in the United States, including a rise in vocal socially conservative factions and "alt-right" hate groups, fueled by leaders such as Mike Pence, who openly condemns and demonizes the LGBTQ community, coming out and realizing one's true self for the Queer Generation hasn't become a walk in the park. The state of current affairs also worries members of the older generations as well, apparent in Lorenzo's words:

We're just gonna—I would like to think we would fight. We'll have to endure it for four to eight years, whatever it may be, I'm hoping it's four. I hope it's four and that's it because Pence scares me even more.

In any such environment, gay men must attempt to separate who they are from the social mores that permeate their lives, reaching a point where they are willing and able to come out. Stephanos, of the AIDS generation, describes his personal experience with this process:

This is when I was like 12 or 13. So, that kind of developed over time. Then, by the time I was in college it was something that I kind of like was fine saying [I'm gay]. And, after actually said it, I almost had a nervous breakdown. I like very quickly like reclaimed it or something, I don't know. Yeah the first time I said it to someone I remember it was a friend of mine who I saw recently, and she remembers because I couldn't even say the word gay—like I was like a—couldn't tell her—she thought I was trying—she thought I was gonna tell her I was in with love her.

As Stephanos intimates, the coming out process is anything but smooth. His words are indicative of the challenges in moving from realization, to internalization, to the full formation of one's gay identity. Along the way, there are many gay men who "become stuck," giving up on the coming out process altogether and finding themselves in heterosexual relationships or married to women, while still harboring same-sex desires.

There are steps forward. There are steps backward. There are years and years of contemplation and perhaps preparation of plans never put into action. Some men are able to go through these stages swiftly, moving forward in the coming out and self-realization process with less resistance. Such good luck comes from myriad factors and circumstances, mostly rooted in a family and culture of love and inclusion. For others, the experience is much more extended, driven by sociopolitical or cultural circumstances, as described throughout this book, or by internal factors. For example, former New Jersey governor Jim McGreevey's aspirations and political ambitions kept him from disclosing his sexual identity for years. In 2004, he got caught up in a scandal that led to him publicly coming out. Though something to be applauded, it only took about 230 years and a scandal for a governor in the United States to acknowledge he was gay. Worse yet, due to the fear that kept him from coming out earlier in his life, knowing full well his chances in politics would likely diminish, McGreevey was forced to live a lie and a double life.

After coming out, however, McGreevey was able to reconcile who he was as a unique individual and a gay man. He left politics behind and went on to join a seminarian program with the Episcopal Church, work at an addiction treatment facility in Newark, New Jersey, and counsel women at a correctional center. The words he spoke when he resigned, "I am a gay American," will never be forgotten and may have even gained further significance in the years since. But there are many other men whose negotiation of their gay identity was never initiated, nor will it ever be. They may maintain same-sex desires, coupled perhaps by same sex behaviors, but never move forward to that next step: openly identifying as gay men and becoming proud members of the LGBTQ community.

BECOMING GAY

"Becoming" a gay man is a unique evolutionary process that we each fashion in our search for identity on our way toward coming out. Of course we are born who we are, but over time we develop an understanding of our sexual identity as gay men. American sexologist Eli Coleman looked at this idea as early as 1982,[9] when he developed a model about this experience, aptly named "Developmental Stages of the Coming-Out Process."

He named the first stage Pre–Coming Out, a period of childhood in which we "learn" through direct and indirect messaging that homosexuality is wrong, just as Juan and Miguel of the Queer Generation were taught by their parents and the communities in which they grew up. Tom, from the Stonewall Generation, described his development as a gay man as a process that occurred over time, also informed in great part by the messages he had heard his entire life:

> [Coming out] peeling the onion to get to the core self, and the authentic, true self, takes a long time, because behavior that is inculcated in me, anyway, from early on in life, and that, that scorn, that dislike of gay—gay people, queers, faggots, whatever you want to call them—was reinforced and reinforced and reinforced over time.

The message that it is wrong to be gay is also informed by societal standards. Seth spoke of this idea eloquently, when he said, "All of our models have been heteronormative. They're, like, how do we fit into that framework when all we're trying to do is discover who we are?" This statement is in line with Coleman's pre–coming out stage, when young people can tell something's different or even "wrong," but are not aware of same-sex feelings yet, as discussed in chapter 1. This idea is exemplified in the words of Miguel, reflecting on his own coming of age:

> There was a sense of effeminate behavior was wrong. So I was taught early on that effeminate behavior from my end was wrong. And my sister was a tomboy at the time, too. So, like, it was, like, she was also given a lot of shit for not acting effeminate. I kind of got all of the social cues from her and her boyfriends and whoever, like, like, to what male essential—what I would call in my adult years male performance. Like, like, I mean, what is it to be masculine. I mean, I would pick that all up from her boyfriend. So, because they were the only dudes who were, like, taking me out to the movies, hanging out with me, spending time with me, like, you know, saying things, like, that was gay. That's not gay. That's . . . and you don't want to be gay.

These early experiences create the foundations for the sense of otherness, and in turn loneliness, which permeates much of our lives.

Coleman's second stage is Coming Out, when gay men acknowledge their feelings, often during adolescence. Young gay men then struggle with having to tell others—a step that Coleman considers essential to self-acceptance. For me, there was a period between 14 and 18 when I silenced these feelings, hoping to get through high school unscathed. Only after high school and once my sexual life with men began did I tell my parents. For Reid, a member of the Queer Generation, his coming out to his mother was akin to my coming out to my father:

> So she found a gay porn magazine under my bed when I was like, 16 years old. LOL, oops. And she was like, "I found something in your room," and that was pretty much the end of that. She was like, "Do you like men?" I was like, "Yeah," and she was like, "Okay." That was the end. That was the end of it. That was literally it. That was the whole coming-out process. Simple, easy, took about eight seconds of my life, and that was it.

And though "that was it" in telling his mother, Reid would not come out to his father until years later—the process was far from complete.

Lorenzo was more methodical in his approach to coming out and acting on his identity. He decided to wait until he turned 21 before his disclosure to his family, worried about their response and uncertain of how they'd react. He was also still hiding the wounds from his early sexual experiences, having been sexually victimized by members of the clergy as a boy:

> I wouldn't do anything before I was 21 because I wanted to go to a bar. I would be in therapy if they ever busted me with a fake I.D. So, I waited. I literally was—turned 21 on February 17. My friends took me to a bar out in Long Island. And they dropped me home around 11:00. I got back in my car and went out to the same town, Island Park, because it was the only gay bar that I knew of. And it was called Cheeks. And I went there; it was a Wednesday night. I think there were like six people in the bar. Two of them or three of them worked there. And that was the moment I came out on the Island. . . . It was kinda rough, um, that telling—telling the people that were closest to me [that I was gay during this early stage/early years of coming out] Um, I did not ever, actually, tell my dad. Um, I had been, you know—because now I had found this community, so, and was legal, I could go into a bar and I didn't have to go home. And I was 21; I didn't have to come home.

And so began Lorenzo's exploration, the next stage of Coleman's model, in which gay men learn how to socialize and meet others who share their sexual interests, since they have likely not yet developed the skills or understanding necessary to having a same-sex relationship. Young gay men are not given guidance on how to love each other or be intimate together, especially when it comes to sex. Same-sex education is not taught in most schools, and there is no one handbook that provides information on all the essential steps of grooming, lubricant, condoms, and other realities they need to know. Few school-based curricula address LGBTQ sociosexual needs, although efforts are underway, particularly in California.[10] The Human Rights Campaign has stated:

> Lesbian, gay, bisexual, transgender, queer and questioning (LGBTQ) youth need and deserve to learn in settings that are inclusive of their experiences and that give them the education necessary to stay safe and healthy. Far too many LGBTQ youth are sitting in classrooms where their teachers and textbooks fail to appropriately address their identities, behaviors and experiences. Nowhere is this absence more clear, and potentially more damaging, than in sex education.[11]

Quite frankly, a gay handbook would have been handy at age 18.

In the exploration stage, many gay men exclusively explore their new social spaces for sex. The illegal bars and clubs of the Stonewall Generation gave way to a multitude of legal bars, clubs, and sex venues where members of the following generation could meet each other freely and without fear of police raids and systematic discrimination, though the fear of AIDS always loomed large. The Queer Generation has transformed these physical spaces into online spaces—though the same behavior exists, the medium is different. These online interactions then develop into physical ones. In this regard, Reid said:

> Right across the street from the church I grew up with, there was a coffee shop that was owned by a gay couple, so every gay person in Grand Rapids would congregate there, so you kind of met people through there. Again, the Internet and social media. I had just gotten my first laptop, and I utilized the WIFI. So I would go there and sit there and talk to people and meet people because that's the kind of personality that I have. I'm just very, "Let's be friends." And then XY was just coming out, too. I don't know if you remember that. It was like Grindr, but even worse. It had, like, a location and a picture and a little blurb where you could type, like, 140 characters or whatever it was at that time. But I was, you know, in high school, and I was 16, and I was gay, and I was a man, so I was horny, and I was curious, and I just wanted to, like, do things and see what happened. [When I had sex] usually it was at their places. We had to be very careful, because—again, it was the Midwest, and a lot of us were only 16 to 18, so we didn't have our own places. I would, like, leave high school and drive up to his place knowing that his parents weren't gonna be home until 6:00 and we would just, like, get it done and that would be that.

The exploration stage for the Stonewall Generation also entailed an artificial dichotomy for many: having sex with other men and still considering themselves straight. Jason describes this idea of duality and staying hidden from his family until life circumstances predicated his disclosure:

> When my mother died, I had to come out to my cousins. That day, when my cousin picked me up—my cousin's husband picked me up—I had to come out to him. I mean, like, they didn't hear it from me. They had not heard from me that I was gay. They knew, you know, "Cousin John in New York, ohhhh," but I never was that close to them. I was not there. . . . We're all animals, and we all get imprinted by our families. So, I sort of put one finger straight, one finger bent, and one is like my father, one is me. And, as one bends down and one goes straight, that's sort of how it evolves into finding your own self, and, uh, and people come to that at different times.

Just as the coming out process remains a constant, the exploration of sexual identity and development also continues to progress over time. Though Thomas came out at age 18, establishing a relationship and exploring his sexuality were intimately connected to being a gay man. In his 30s, he and his partner entered into a "trouple," a three-member "couple," while the AIDS epidemic was beginning:

> So, Ben met Mark. They did not have sex, but Mark was a med student at the time, and Ben invited him to come to New York and stay with us. And Mark would say, "Oh, no, I can't, I'm too busy," but Ben would convince him and say, "Mark, there'll be a ticket"—he was a man of the grand gesture. "Mark, there'll be a ticket waiting for you at, you know, the counter. You come for the weekend." Um, and so, he did, and we all became good friends. Now, in the beginning of that relationship, there was sex. The three of us, uh, had a sexual relationship for a while. Interestingly, I think, um, Mark, uh, was infected by Ben. I'm pretty sure. And that was back in—shit, was it 1982?

In Coleman's model, after the exploration period, the next stage is first relationships. It is overly simplistic to assume, however, that gay men come out, have endless casual encounters, and then proceed to establish relationships—one and done. As noted in the words of Tom above, sexual exploration is often tied to relationships, even as the coming out process continues. Coleman's misunderstanding may have been shaped by his own life experience, having been born in 1948 and coming of age prior to 1969. He argued that a period of sexual experimentation may be superseded by a need for intimacy and connection, but in fact these can certainly, and often do, function together.

This was clearly the case for Wilson, whose sexual exploration was bound to his complex first relationship with Ronnie in the late 1950s, a particularly challenging time for two black gay men:

When we hooked up, he worked at this insurance company. [It was 1956], I worked [there] from March to September. So, I met him then. Ronnie played bass in his school orchestra. He went to Boys High, in Brooklyn. It was—at that time, it was a very good school. And he played bass on weekends, sometimes he would get a gig, you know. But it wasn't a vocation, it was more an avocation. And so, he put a card on my desk, saying he could play bass, he was for hire and all like that. Because he knew I was interested in music. But I know this was his way of breaking the ice. So, we had a holiday. I think it was Memorial Day. Back then . . . whatever day it fell on, that's the day you were off. And this week, it fell on a Friday that year. May 30th was Friday. That's Memorial Day, so the office was closed. But what they decided was you could choose. You could come to work a half a day Memorial Day and have July 4th off. So I chose to work Memorial Day, and so did he. So, the office is now half—half empty, and we're the only black guys—ones, because the other black guys wanted to, you know, have Memorial Day off or something. So, he says let's go to lunch. And I'm thinking, oh my, he's going to take me to lunch, you know. But I'm—he's black and lives in Brooklyn, Caribbean, you know. And he was sort of built nice and—but very pleasant. And so, I'm thinking, okay, where are we going? We're sitting and we're talking, and he tells me that he's got a girlfriend, and they're high school sweethearts, and blah-blah. And that he's saving money because he's going to get engaged—Thanksgiving he's planning—now, this is Memorial Day, right? May, at the end of May. And he's planning to buy the engagement ring. That's what he's saving his money for, because somewhere around Thanksgiving, he's—he would have enough money to buy the ring and propose. So, I'm thinking, oh, isn't that sweet? You know, I didn't think—so, he says to me, "What are you doing this weekend?" I said, "Well, I don't know." He says, "Well, I got a gig, but he said, "I won't be over—finished work till midnight. And he said, can you—would you be willing to come and we could have a drink after work? Because I'll have some money. I'll get paid. But I want you to—but you have to—you know, I don't get paid until midnight when it's over. Would you be willing to wait?" I said yes. So, he said come to the corner of Park Avenue and 51st Street or something. I'm standing on the corner, under the street lamp, and I'm waiting, and I'm saying this guy, now, if he doesn't show, and all this. And sure enough, about 30 minutes later, I stood there and waited. I see him coming up the block with this bass, because it's got a wheel on it, and he's got it over his shoulder with the wheel—you know, it has a cover zipped—that he zipped up. And—so I could tell, I said that must be him with the bass.

So he walks up and he says, "Um, I don't feel like carrying this bass around." And so, Ronnie lives in Brooklyn. He says, let's get a cab and go home, and then we can go to a bar. You know, go have a drink or something. We get to his house. His older siblings are gone, so there's only him and his younger brother, and I'm not sure where his sister is, who's—you know, the one—it's only the one girl, right? So— but, so he now has the whole ground floor. And when I walk in, I say, oh, boy, he's got things all neat, and—and there's a bottle. I—so, I mean, this is all hindsight. I said, he had no intention of us going to a bar. He was going to bring me to his house and fuck the shit out of me—which is what he did that night. Oh my God. I was shocked. I had no idea he was interested, you know? And that's—so—and it was so, no, we can't say anything at work. I said no problem.

That Sunday morning, I get—we get up, and he says I'll give you cab fare to get home with. And so, I go get ready to leave, and he opens the door, and he looks at me and he says, I don't love you. I love my girl. And I said where did that come from, you know? I—okay, bye, you know.

Though Wilson had been with other men, his experience with Ronnie had been different. Not only had their sexual encounter taken him by surprise, but so did Ronnie's subsequent doting:

So, he calls. Did you get home alright? Can I come see you? It was terrific—our first sex that night. So, he—and he wanted to do it again. So, I said okay. So—and my aunt and uncle were completely, uh, okay with [me having guests]. So, he started coming to my house. And I would say, listen, don't be confused. Let me tell you what I know. Now, big time—I'm 18, but I say, I've been—so, you know, I tell him, look, get married, this would be much easier for you. I have many, many guys that I know who've married and whenever they feel like, they go and do it, and come back home to their wife and family. This has been going on for centuries. You know, so don't feel bad. Get comfortable with yourself. If you love this girl, you want to marry her, go ahead and get married. And any time you want to see me, you know, I'm okay with this. But you know, I'm going on, because, you know.

Wilson saw the relationship moving toward one that was more purely physical, one in which Ronnie could lead a double life, not unlike many members of the Stonewall years, never coming out and openly developing his gay identity. But their budding intimacy, emotional and physical, didn't end there:

So, then, he says, I'll get you—I'll help you look for an apartment. You can move away from your aunt and uncle.

So, that July, I found an apartment on Lexington Avenue between 31st and 32nd. There was a gay bar called the 32, which was on 32nd Street between Madison and Park, a white, a white gay bar. So, this one night, I come home, 4:00 the bar closes, and I had to get up and go to work. There he is, standing outside my door. And he says, "This is not going to work. I've been standing here waiting for you." I said, "Well, why didn't you—" I said, "You knew where I was. You know I go to the bar to—" See, he didn't want to go in a gay bar. And so, he's standing there. It's winter, and he's angry as all outdoors. I mean, I'm not—I'm getting a little nervous, because I haven't seen him like this. The fuck you doing in this bar? Where—who you been with? This—what shit—da-da-da-da-da-da. Come on up-stairs. Upstairs. He kind of grabs me, slams me up against the wall. Uh-uh, this shit is not going to work. I don't know what the fuck you doing and who you been messing with. I want you myself. It's the only way this can happen is we get an apartment together. What? Wait a minute. Aren't you—a little like the cart be-fore the horse or something, you know? You haven't asked me and you know, you don't—I'm telling you. And sure enough, by—this is—like I say, this is winter. It's cold. So, I don't know if it's even after Christ—after Christmas, but that April is when we moved to 88th Street.

At this interview Wilson brought copies of the love letters he and Ronnie exchanged during that period of time, which were bound in leather books. My heart melted.

Sixty years later, establishing relationships for young gay men is in some ways just as complex, conflated with the biases of race and class that men of color frequently experience. For Miguel, sexual exploration and the search for a relationship led him to social spaces where race, gender, and sexuality are more fluid, allowing people to fully realize who they are, while rejecting the white male cisgender, privileged hypermasculine characteristics that too often dominate gay culture. His story is also characterized by the on-going coming out process, which continued as he developed a deeper un-derstanding of his sexual and gender fluidity and place within the LGBTQ community:

So I found, myself really in conflict with the queer community here in New York. I found, like, I was a gay man in a city full of gay men but I couldn't connect with any of them. None of them understood what I was doing. Like, there was, like, a team of Chelsea gay men who just didn't understand my, like, socioeconomic back-ground. Like, they just, like, "being poor, what's that like?" Like, I, I couldn't con-nect with them. And then there was a whole team of Brooklyn gays who were all these, like, ex-pats who had also come from, like, wealthy, um, very easy lives. I felt like a lot of their coming out stories whenever we related was just, like, yeah, I told my mom one day that, you know, I was gay, and she was fine with it. I was like, what the fuck? Like, I didn't have any kind of relationship with, with specifically gay white cis men. Like, I couldn't connect with them. But even men of color were having—I was having a hard time connecting with. I ended up finding out that I was just, like, well maybe I'm queer.

So there was a vibrant kind of queer community that was sort of growing, uh, be-tween, like, men of color and black men that I was sort of being like, you know, I, this is—I feel more at home here. And it was also like trans men and, you know, trans women, and, you know, lesbian women, and, like, people from across the spectrum. And it felt like—I was like, this is exactly where I want to be. Like, this is, like, I can't be in a room with only gay men. I have to be in a room that's as diverse as how I feel inside. So I was like, I have to do this.

Integration is the final stage of Coleman's model, a period in which a person's public and private identities merge into one and are shaped by growing up into adulthood. Though it may not be what Coleman intended, in realty this stage is one that persists throughout life as all members of the LGBTQ community seek to integrate and make sense of who they are, fusing their cultural, racial, ethnic, sexual, cognitive, spiritual, economic, and professional identities. This portfolio of identifies is similar to American psychologist Howard Gardner's portfolio of multiple intelligences, in so much as people possess different intelligences and call on specific ones depending on circumstances and cognitive tasks.

So too, gay identity and other identities emerge in varying ways in different environments—it is no wonder that the coming out process therefore continues in perpetuity for most. Integration is more than a stage, it is a condition in which LGBTQ people never hide nor cover their gay identity. This identity may not be the most prominent one in a given situation but it is also never negated—it is, as stated at the beginning of the chapter, part of being. In the words of 23-year-old Yasar:

For me, it means living my truth and um being able to navigate honestly in a society where heterosexism is so prominent in most cultures, basically all cultures— and yeah, I guess just being able to be different and—yeah, be different and live honestly.

Stephanos, age 42, also spoke of this sense of wholeness accompanying his understanding of what it means to be gay:

I know one point meant it was like a word [gay] to identify at the very least a set of feelings that I had that I couldn't put a name to, or that I did put a name to in, but couldn't like compartmentalize myself about.

And for 66-year-old Jim integration was central to his coming out and how he thought of his gay identity:

I'm proud, I'm out, and there's no hidden parts of me; it has to do with um maybe my way of looking at relationships. Maybe a way of relating to people. But what is it like to be a gay man, doesn't—doesn't resonate all that much, for me. I've been out for a very long time and so it's sort of part of the fiber.

Across generations, all gay men seek the freedom to express who we are, and a consistent part of that expression is our need to come out again and again. For some, it can be exhausting, but it also gives us an opportunity to display our pride in our sexuality and in the people we have become. We have only gotten to this point in our history through the decades of fighting for LGBTQ rights. Only through the coming out process can we integrate our gay identity into our whole being, owning and honoring the identity that some are stuck searching for their whole lives. It becomes our journey, personally and collectively, and it is the work of achieving our truth.

FINAL THOUGHTS

The conditions around coming out shape our life trajectories, our health, and our well-being. The process, though similar for many, does not necessarily occur in a fixed lock-step pattern—far from it. There is wide variation in coming out and how it shapes our identity development. For some, there is never even a realization of their true selves. While there is an orderly developmental process at the foundation of gay identity formation, as seen in the Coleman model, the patterns are never fully predictable, especially over time. In some ways it's similar to how children acquire language skills or how adolescents merge into adulthood.

Who or what we strive to be, and some day become, relies on our generation and who we are as people, including where we live in the world, and when; how we're raised; and the experiences we have at a young age. Our sexual, social, emotional, political, spiritual, and cognitive lives all play a role and intersect throughout our lifetimes. During that process, most gay men realize that they are still coming out, even to themselves, as attested to by Tom in the opening of this chapter: "Every time I experience internal homophobia, I realize that's a place where I haven't come out yet, where I feel uncomfortable just being who I am. You know, I haven't truly become comfortable with me as a person, the authentic me." We all move from a period of uncertainty of who we were as children into a lifelong quest to integrate our gay identity into all aspects of our lives, coming out again and again, confronting challenges within families, social circles, and society itself. These experiences are the ones that define our coming out stories and make us who we are.

REFERENCES

1. Williams R. People coming out as gay at younger age, research shows. *The Guardian* 2010.
2. George Michael comes out on CNN (1998). CNN Entertainment 2016.

3. Afanador R. Interview: Sam Smith on coming out, and *The Thrill of It All. The Times* 2017.
4. Queerty Staff. Can we please come up with a new way to say "coming out"? *Queerty* 2010.
5. Nicolosi J, Byrd AD, Potts RW. Beliefs and practices of therapists who practice sexual reorientation psychotherapy. *Psychol Rep.* 2000;86(2):689–702.
6. Brook B. Claims parishioners were "screamed at" by anti-same-sex marriage priest who demanded his flock all vote no. *News.com.au* 2017.
7. Minton HL, McDonald GJ. Homosexual identity formation as a developmental process. *J Homosex.* 1983;9(2–3):91–104.
8. Habermas T, Bluck S. Getting a life: the emergence of the life story in adolescence. *Psychol Bull.* 2000;126(5):748–769.
9. Coleman E. Developmental stages of the coming out process. *J Homosex.* 1981;7(2–3):31–43.
10. Schaub M. California will be the first state to use LGBT-inclusive history textbooks in schools. *Los Angeles Times* 2017.
11. Human Rights Campaign. A call to action: LGBTQ youth need inclusive sex education. https://www.hrc.org/resources/a-call-to-action-lgbtq-youth-need-inclusive-sex-education. Accessed July 8, 2018.

CHAPTER 4
Telling

Every gay man who has managed to achieve some level of self-actualization and identity integration has a story, or numerous stories, of coming out. These stories are often complex and colorful, painful and perpetuating, and ultimately always life altering. As discussed in the previous chapter, coming out is an ongoing process, but there are moments that define the experience in which family and close friends learn about the sexual identities of the gay men in their lives, whether told directly, found out accidentally, or intimated but never spoken.

Volume upon volume could be written about coming out to different people in various situations—whether to colleagues or friends, at work or at school—but the most important people to whom we speak our truth are our families, and in particular, our parents. This event is often the strongest in shaping the lives of young gay men, given the attachment children have with their parents, and one of the most challenging aspects of gay identity development.[1] It is also an integral step in the realization and actualization of gay identity, in the maintenance and growth of self-esteem,[2] and in the ability for a gay couple to establish a healthy and meaningful relationship.[3]

In the end, the motivation to feel complete and whole is one of the main drivers behind gay men disclosing their sexual identity to their parents.[4] Jeremy emphasized this importance:

> Once I did that [came out] and everybody was more accepting it was—like I said, my dad's just changed for the better. It was weird. And just being able to be myself around my family. Because that's kind of where I used to be, you know, I was—I was always myself around my family, but then, when I decided to accept to me that I was gay, I wanted to be—I wanted them to know that too. And I wanted to be okay with coming around and them knowing that. Then me bringing, you know, friends over that are gay, or a boyfriend.

Though coming out is a personal experience that contributes to identity development, a psychological reality with wide variation for gay men,[5] it is also a communal reality.[6-8] The relationships of those within the family and the person's social circles are also affected by this revelation, in some cases precipitating a crisis that needs to be resolved.[9] For many parents, this new knowledge is often immediately experienced as mourning and loss.[10] However, as with most losses, these feelings subside in their impact over time.

Tom articulately described this communal phenomenon:

> Coming out is not just an experience of the person who is coming out. Coming out is an experience of the parents. You know, they have to go through a process, and that's what so many gay men don't understand, is that, yeah, you're coming out, and there's certain kinds of trauma, whatever you want to call it, associated with that, and that is a process, but your parents have to come out with you. They need to, um, adjust to this whole way of a lifestyle that they hadn't—I'll say, had no idea that you were living, and they need to make an adjustment to it, and I think a lot of gay men fail their parents.

Many parents in the United States know little about the lesbian, gay, bisexual, transgender, and queer (LGBTQ) community or what being gay truly entails. A large number of them are also embedded in a dominantly heteronormative, intolerant culture, creating the crux of the problem we experience as we attempt to fully realize our identities. In fact, professor Adital Ben-Ary, the head of University of Haifa's Center for Research and Study of the Family, has demonstrated that the processes associated with coming out for children were made easier when parents were educated prior to their kids' vocalization of sexual identity.[11] With the ushering in of the Queer Generation, more research has also been focused on how sexual disclosure plays out for different races and ethnicities as well. It has been reported that there are no racial or ethnic differences in the age one initially comes out, but people of color were less likely to be out to their parents.[12]

The emotional vicissitude of many parents in response to their son's disclosure is common, fraught with feelings of attachment with their child and coupled with confusion, concern, and on plenty of occasions, anger and rejection. Such reactions align with the need for parents to readjust their understanding of the course of their child's life[13] and most come to tolerate or accept their child's sexual orientation in time.[10] To be clear, tolerance and acceptance are not synonymous and should not be conflated. The healthiest and most beneficial resolution for any young gay men coming out is when their parents accept them and realign familial expectations and structures as necessary. This process is not always easy, as both parents and their children must learn how to relate to one another all over again, as if they are truly getting to know each other for the first time. In doing so, they reestablish and redefine their relationships.

Just as there is no lockstep pattern for coming out, there is also no predetermined manner in which all parents can be expected to react, but research indicates that parental attitudes are progressing. A Pew Research Institute report published in 2015[14] found that 57% of parents would not be upset if they learned their child was gay. Despite this high proportion, 39% noted that they would be upset in some way, with 17% reporting they would be very upset. So even though members of the Queer Generation in the United States seem to be comfortable coming out at a younger age than their predecessors, they still need to navigate the emotions and psychosocial burdens that are likely to arise and could potentially affect their health and well-being at the time or later on in life. No matter the generation, telling your parents about the most intimate part of yourself, one that you might not yet even fully comprehend, never gets easier. The interviewees' stories attest to that fact, but they also attest to the resilience and fortitude of these men, and the ability to find one's self among the words spoken or written.

TELLING PARENTS

Before Emilio came out to his parents, he began by telling some of his siblings. Though no small feat in itself, he knew that disclosing that he was both gay and HIV-positive to his parents would be more difficult, and he decided that a phone call, as he had done with some of his brothers and sisters, wasn't how he wanted to approach his mom and dad. He planned to gather his thoughts, write a letter, send it to them, and then visit them in person to talk it all over.

> So I decided it's time to come out. So I came out to the siblings. They were accepting. I told them I was gonna tell Mom and Dad. I told them about the letter situation, and I would go visit them [our parents] in Buffalo and have a conversation with them.

When Emilio got to Buffalo, his parents had already read the following note:

> Dear Mom and Dad. Boy, I don't even know where to begin with this letter. It probably is the hardest thing that I will ever have to write. And I hope that someday you will understand why I am doing this. Because this is so important to me. I have decided to type it rather than write it. First of all, I want to thank you so much for being wonderful parents. Not only have you both come from different countries and

learned to speak English—the English language, but you have also done so much more. You have raised six bright, and loving children, you have also ensured our success, by teaching us—all of us to be proud, independent, and to have love for each other, no matter what. The strength of love is the reason I can no longer deny the truth. I want you to know me and love me for who I really am. Secondly, I want you to know, at this point in my life, I have never been happier or healthier. This is the first time in my life that I can actually love myself. What I am trying to tell you is that I am gay. I am sorry if I have lied to you about this matter, but this is something I had to figure out for myself. Although you may think this news is shocking, it may be part of—uh–it has been part of me for my entire life. I might seem different to you now, but in reality, I'm the same son you have always had. I'm not telling you this to hurt or embarrass you, but simply because I love you. Mom and Dad, I did date Nina Tavares for almost three years, and yes, I did propose to her. The only reason I went through with all of this was because that was the way I thought life was supposed to be. I was never really happy back then. I always thought maybe I could even start up a relationship with Karen. I'm telling you these things because I want you to know that I'm very happy, and I must continue on with my life. Mom and Dad, you have been through so many hardships. Both of you survived World War II; Mom, you lived through the Spanish Civil War. I know that unless you were not honest with yourselves and the ones you loved, you could not have gone through these experiences. You both have so much integrity. You also have said that you will love your children, no matter what. And I hope that you would love me, even though I'm also HIV positive. This means that I've been exposed to the AIDS virus. There is a chance that I might progress to AIDS and there also is a chance that I may not. I must remind you that at this point in my life, I'm very healthy. I am asymptomatic. I've been on AZT for one year, and I'm currently using a new drug, which is in trial. I hope I will be a long term survivor of AIDS. With your love and support, that is a definite possibility. Mom and Dad, you both have your own health problems. Dad had a great recovery from Hodgkin's Disease; and Mom, you had your heart to worry about. My position is now pretty much the same as yours. I want you to know that [my siblings and their spouses] have all shown great support for me. I don't know about [another male sibling] yet because I just sent him the letter. Well, Mom and Dad. Where do we go from here? I hope that you will not make yourselves, yourselves sick from worrying about me. Once again, let me tell you, I'm very happy and healthy now. And that the reason that I've decided to tell you at this time, I think it is better that you find out like this rather than if I happen to really get sick, perhaps even die. I want you to know that I will get colds and flu, just like everybody else. At the present time, I think it's best for us to continue our relationship. The only difference now is that you know me a lot better. The reason I wrote this letter before coming to visit you was so that you could have some time to think about things. [Female sibling] will also be informed about the letter, so if you need to talk to her, please call her. If you even want to give me a call, please call me, too. Remember, all I want to do is—all I want you to know is that I love you very much and hope we can let our relationship grow from here. If I have to live my life over again, I wouldn't change a thing. I'll see you on Saturday. Love.

This incredible, heartfelt letter was followed by his parents' concern, but mostly about Emilio's HIV status, given that they were both health professionals:

> You know, they were very like, really, really concerned. My dad, I don't really think had an issue with me being gay. He never said anything. I never felt judgment from him. He was kind—concerned about the HIV part. But you know. But my mom was like, "Oh, my God. You're gonna die. And la, la, la, la, la." I was like, "No, I'm not gonna die." And I just—about calming her down. And then she's like, "What did I do wrong? Why are you gay?" . . . for me it was because my dad was nonreligious and my mother was strictly, really strictly religious. I think that's where the basis of that came from for my parents.

Jeremy, of the Queer Generation, also first approached other family members before his parents. His emotional and sexual lives as a gay man had emerged throughout high school, shifting from years of covering his sexuality by dating women, and culminating in a need to come out. He, too, had a methodology to his disclosure, starting by telling extended family:

> I told, kind of, like, all the cousins. Just, like, I think it was through the phone call, or through—and I'm just—and I was just saying I'm—I'm accepting it more now, so I'm telling you guys. So it was the cousins. And then they told their moms, and stuff like that, which were my aunts and uncles, but with my permission. Because I kind of wanted—I just—my parents were last because I just didn't know how they were going to take it. And so it took some time, I guess, for me to tell them. It took, like, maybe a month or two. I told them, like, around July. I told my mom. So, my dad was basically the last person to find out because I just didn't know how he was going to take it. And, I just—I don't know. I—I—I didn't know if he was going to accept me after that. And things like that. So I told my mom to tell my dad.

At the time, Jeremy had just started his first same-sex relationship, which acted as the spark for his identity revelation. He knew that coming out would potentially enable him to develop a fuller relationship with his new partner, Sonny:

> So Sonny was the one that—he helped me. He helped me come out to my parents, and all that, because he had already been out to his parents. Him and I, kind of, grew up, like, I would say, from teenage to adulthood. Like, a lot of our relationship, we were, like, together for most of that. So I feel like I grew up with him. Like, we both grew up into adults together. And we were there for each other a lot. He was there through that. I mean, he stuck around, even after I contracted that [HIV].

I was, like, coming out of the shower. So I had been dating Sonny for, since, like, May. You know, this new found love, like, that was different from dating girls. It was, like, and the sex was great, which was different from having sex with girls. So throughout those three months, I had always told my mom, like, oh, I'm going to go see this girl that I'm talking to, when it was really Sonny.

So then, that's, kind of, how I told her. I was, like, "Well, the girl that I've been seeing is really a guy." And she was, like, "What are you talk—" she just couldn't believe it. She's like, "What are you trying to say?" And she—same thing. She thought I was, like, joking with her. And I'm, like, "No, I'm telling you the truth. Like, I'm gay. And it's a guy." And then she was just, like, kind of in shock. Um, I was going somewhere, so I kind of did it on purpose, I think. Saying it to where I was leaving right after.

And then she told my dad. And he was, like, we didn't talk about it for, like, a whole week. And he was, like, moping around. Like, very depressed. You could see that he was, like, crying, and things like that. Like, I don't know. He was just going through it for, like, a whole week.

Then he finally came up to me in my room and was, like, "Well, you're still my son, you know. I'll accept you no matter what." And it was very short. It wasn't really like we spoke about it much. But then I remember sometime throughout the year that my mom was, I don't know. Because they were talking to my aunt a lot, one of my younger aunts that was, like, one of my really good friends. She's also one of—was somebody that I came out with, like, when I—when I came out to— when I came out to my cousins. I told her too. But they were talking to her a lot, I guess because she was the younger aunt, and we used to hang out a lot. And, like, they were trying to talk to her about, like, for me to see a doctor. Nothing was ever brought up to me. But, they were, like, talking to my aunt about this. Like, they wanted me, maybe, to see a doctor. They thought it was a stage. They were—they'd just never been confronted with a situation like that. And I didn't think they ever thought their son would be gay. And—but eventually, it just kind of all blew over.

Reid, another member of the Queer Generation, planned to come out to his dad via text message. After having come out to most of his friends around age 13 and to his mother when he was 16, somewhat accidentally, as mentioned in the previous chapter, Reid prepared to tell his dad about his sexual identity. After telling his mom, he realized the significance of the act, and not just in his own life, but in the lives of all gay men:

I don't think it matters what generation you grew up in. As a gay man, every gay man has to come out to their parents, and it's always like a big thing. It doesn't matter if you're 60 or if you're 14. You have to sit down and have that conversation. I think—because your parents raised you from, like, the ground up, right? And I feel like they know you more than you know you in a sense, because they've watched you from, like, a little child all the way up to whatever you are now. And if you can't be completely open and honest with your parents, you're not being open and honest with yourself at the end of the day. And I feel like your parents are kind of like that hurdle, where you're like, to me, that's when I think I fully accepted the fact that I was gay, when I came out to my mom. Like, that was a big hurdle, and I was like, "Okay, like, this is done. Now I don't have to act a certain way or pretend to be somebody else or dress a certain way when I'm around her. I can just be who I want to be."

Every gay man finds his own way of coming out to his parents, relying on the social-emotional tools with which he is most comfortable, as a means of creating the psychological space to allow his identity to continue to develop. Reid pointed out this fact:

I don't think there's a right or wrong way to come out. I feel like everybody does it their own way, but I think at some point that you do need to have a conversation with your parents, because eventually, you're going to hit a point where you're gonna want to start dating and maybe you're gonna bring, like, somebody home with you for holidays or whatnot, and there's nothing more uncomfortable when you're like, "LOL, surprise! Here it is!"

While Reid believes the process of coming out is significant, he is also critical of his generation's abuse of social media in telling their stories. Although he considers social media as a helpful tool for gay men, one which he uses plenty, in his view it is a tool that must be managed:

Especially in our generation, where social media's everywhere and you always have to; like, when people come out now, they make a big fucking deal, and they upload it to YouTube, and they have like five million views, and they're super dumb and obnoxious. I don't think it needs to be to that extreme. It said something to me as an individual when I finally came out to my mom. You know, it was a big thing.

After telling his mother, it would be another 8 years before Reid would disclose his sexual identity to his father directly, although he had done so indirectly for years through his posts to social media, which have become central to his identity and image as a gay man:

My dad I came out to through text message, actually when I was 24. So that was kind of recently. I had come home. I've always wanted to work in the music industry and I had just graduated, and I had moved to Chicago and I was like, "Oh, things are starting to happen," and I started to become kind of a public figure. I had started a YouTube page and posted a coming out video that ended up getting close to 13 million views before I finally took it down. . . . But my dad was friends with me on Facebook. He had seen the videos I posted, because I would post them and then I would post the link to my status. So I know he had seen it, and I had just come home from Christmas, and I was on my way back. I was on the Megabus back to Chicago, and I was like—I think I still have the text message, actually.

FORCING THE CONVERSATION

Though some choose to take a methodical approach to coming out, it's also common for mini crises of sorts to aid in initiating the conversation. Yasar's experience, for example, was spontaneous, precipitated by circumstance. Raised in a traditional Ghanaian Pentecostal family, he knew his parents' reaction would be far from supportive. One night, after having a few drinks, he decided then and there that he couldn't wait any longer. As a member of the Queer Generation, he understood the sense of empowerment that would come with making the statement "I am gay" to his parents and how it may help him in better understanding himself as well. The time had come: he needed to get the words out, even if that meant drunk dialing his dad:

> So it was 9:45 and I take two shots of peach Burnett's vodka. Not my glory days. But um yeah I upgraded from that. But anyways. Two shots, 9:45. Yeah, so. I called my dad and I tell him that I'm gay. Starts off with I asked him if he loved me and he said yes. And then I told him that I was gay and his reaction was basically just like saying wow. He just kept saying wow. And he had nothing else to say. I was like okay. So then he got off the phone with me, I think he asked me like, "How did you think [I'd react?]"—something like that. I can't remember my response. But then he got off the phone with me, but him and my mom they were helping my brother, because his car was on the side of the road on the side of the highway. . . . So basically I get off the phone with him and then my mom calls me like five minutes—not even five minutes, like two minutes [later]. And the first thing she tells me, she tells me she's like crying. She's like "Yasar don't kill me." I was like "Yo what are you talking about?" And she just kept on saying that and then she started crying and um she's just like "You're going to hell," like all this stuff, "I don't want you to go to hell I want you to go to heaven," and all this other stuff. And we were arguing for about ten minutes. I was feeling horrible. Like that's, I mean, like I knew that was coming but I just never—it wasn't a great conversation.

Yasar's parents' solution to their son's "gay problem" differed from Lorenzo's and Jim's, whose parents sent them to psychotherapy when they came out. Instead, they believed Yasar's sexual identity salvation would be rooted in the words of god:

But after I came out, my dad—I was more worried about my dad because he has more power over me you know; like he tried to get me out of school at one point. But yeah, like on Sunday, every Sunday, he would call me and tell me off and tell me that, "You shouldn't be gay." So it was like at 1:00 when he gets out from church, so I'm like—he was kinda cool with it, or he didn't necessarily have a negative reaction when I told him. So it wasn't until Sunday until he felt the nerve to tell me how he felt. And it was every Sunday after. So he just felt so compelled, he got the will of god or whatever and um yea, just told me, just like told me off. And also it goes back to the internalized, well basically homophobia and the cultural aspect of that because a lot of Ghanaians also say that being gay is not African or just like the narrative, a construct of the Pentecostal church and then they're manipulating it to fit that anti-Western narrative of being gay is bad.

At the opposite end of the age spectrum is Wilson, who, now 78 years old, came out to his mother only after being prodded. His coming out story is a complex tale of rejection intimately overturned by love, acceptance, and pride. While a teenager, Wilson began dating an older white man named Niles, whom he had met at work and who became a big part of Wilson's life. Though he didn't hide this relationship from his family, he also hadn't openly explained it either. Over time, his mother started to suspect that Niles was more than just a customer at the soda counter where Wilson worked:

So, I came home from school one day. My mother had an alcoholism problem, and she had been drinking. Now, she's with my new dad, and she'd been drinking. And she said, "Come here." Now, see, I had met Niles and he was coming to visit me in my all-black neighborhood. Here comes this white dude to my house, and here the two of us leave together, and he's older than I am, and here we go, you know? I hadn't even paid it one rabbit-ass bit of mind, and my mother says to me, "Come here. I want to talk to you." I'm gonna—"Yes." So, she says, "Are you a sissy?" I said, "Well, if you mean am I a homosexual, yes." You know, because I am and I looked right at her. She said, "Well, I wanted to know, because the neighbors are talking. They're asking me questions. You are my child, and whatever it is that you want to be in life, I want you to be the best that there is. I'm asking you this because I want to know what I should say when other people come to me with this." And I don't remember her exact words, I wish I could, but she so much as said, "Then I can tell them to kiss my ass and kiss my child's ass," you know? I mean, that was—I don't remember what she said, but that was her attitude. You are my child, and if anybody says anything about you to me, I will cuss them—call them a couple of motherfuck—I mean, but you know, that wasn't her language, but that's what she meant.

Though Wilson's mother was accepting and open, his father had a harder time adjusting to this new reality, as shown in this confrontation over pictures Wilson had put up in his room:

Okay. So, this is 10th grade. 11th grade, I come home one day. My father says, "Take them goddamn faggots off my wall." This is my room. I'm working. My mother forced me to give her—give them money. I thought that was a big—something we have—mother, how could you, in my own—mother, take my money? I'm so glad she taught me that, right? You know, if I'm bringing $30.00 home, $30.00 a week home, which was a lot of money then, I had to give her $6.00. She said she wanted $6.00 of this $30.00. So, I'm paying rent, I told him. "These are my walls, I want them down, take them"—you know. And we had this huge fight, you know. He said, "I'm sick and tired of this. Take them down. I said take them faggots off the wall." So I said, "Well, I'm not gonna stay here." I went upstairs and packed my bags. I called my mother's father, see, whom I had lived with, and told him to come and get me. Well, he and my father were close. I mean, they got along very well. He really didn't know what it was about, but when he came and I got in the car, I told him that we had just had this fight. And I don't remember what I said to my grandfather about the gay—you know, I don't know how I got that in, because I hadn't come out to him. You know, he's older and a minister and. So he said, "Boy, you can't stay with me. Come on," he said. "Let me think about things"—because he wanted to talk to my dad, you know. My grandfather then took me to his house and told me, "You can't stay here. I'll get one of my parishioners." They had a house, and she rented—she had three—a house with maybe three bedrooms. She had a bedroom, and she rented out the other two, because she lived alone and she was aging, and this was a little extra money for her. So—because I was working, my grandfather told her that I could pay the weekly rent for the room, and that's how it happened. So, that June, the end of the semester, I came home from school, and my landlady said—I went upstairs, and my landlady said—come—calling me from downstairs. "Come downstairs, baby. Come downstairs. Somebody's here to see you." So, I said alright. I came downstairs, and she said, "He's outside in the car." So, I got outside, and there's my father, sitting in the car. And he says, "Come down here. Get in the car." He says, "I'm very proud of you." He says, "You've stayed in school, you got good grades," blahdy-blahdy-blahdy-blah. "But I want you to finish high school and the only way I can be certain of that is if you are under my roof. I want you to go upstairs, get all of your shit, and bring it down here. I'm taking you home."

Similar to Wilson's mom, Seth's parents had suspicions of their son's sexual identity as well. Coming of age during the AIDS generation, Seth's sexual promiscuity started early in adolescence and, like Wilson, eventually led him to engage in sex with older men. One such situation precipitated his coming out to his father and stepmother when he was 16. Evidence suggests that parental reactions are also shaped by socioeconomic status. This was certainly the case for Seth, whose father and stepmother, both of whom had high levels of education, were more concerned about his emotional safety than his sexual identity:

> So I left there [a three-way with an older couple] and went home, and you know, it was already kind of late, and my folks were wondering where I was and there was another issue that they were angry about that they wanted to confront me with, and we were all getting kind of angry, and they wanted to know where I was, and so I kind of spit it out at them in a very vitriolic way that I had just, you know, fucked these two guys, and you know, and they were older than me, and um, I just had my first three-way, and like really shocking; and that was the point, I think. And, um, so, this is my dad and stepmother, and they said, you know it was after they took a breath and looked at each other, they said, "Okay, you know, none of that matters, you are our son, we love you; this isn't all that unexpected, but you're also 15, and um, we forbid you to see men who are over 18." Because it's against the law, it's rape, and they really wanted to instill this idea of—that I was—of the potential danger. And of course, that was like, I wasn't expecting—I wasn't expecting, one, the very positive or at least the acceptance—My folks, my family have always been incredibly accepting, liberal, yeah, we wouldn't—I don't think—I couldn't imagine them being otherwise. So I guess I was just looking for—spoiling for a fight, you know, just in general. But the idea of them rejecting me because I was gay, I guess that didn't even occur to me, actually. I didn't expect the restriction.

Tom, of the Stonewall Generation, lived an open life as a gay man with everyone—except his parents. Though he had come out at age 18 to his friends, and even maintained an adult relationship with his partner Ben for years, he didn't disclose his sexual identity to his parents until he was 35. They had been aware that Ben was Tom's roommate but the matter of sexuality went unspoken, although likely understood: "My mother didn't know I was gay, except she'd send us matching nightshirts for Christmas."

Tom's fear of his father—a high school teacher, principal, and football/basketball coach father, who had been physically abusive to his mother and generally prone to violence—precluded his disclosure at a younger age. Ben's illness, and eventual death from complications of AIDS, served as a catalyst for Tom—if it hadn't been for the surrounding circumstances, he may never have told them. Like many families, his was thrown into a state of chaos and a period of inevitable but imperfect adjustment:

> 1985 was when Ben started getting ill, and when I went to tell them. I had hired a man to take care of Ben because he needed care sort of around the clock. His name was Gino, he was a lovely Brazilian guy who was gay, and I had a car at the time, and I said, "Gino, we're gonna drive to my parents' house in Pennsylvania." I called them first, and I said, "Would you like me to come for lunch on Sunday?" And they

said, "Sure, why not?" So, we got there, and I said to Gino, "Now, turn the car around in the driveway, and keep it running," and I went in and had lunch with my parents. During lunch, I didn't have the courage . . . but afterwards, when we were sitting in the living room, I said, "Oh, there's something I have to tell you," and I said, "I'm gay." And the first words out of my father's mouth were, "Do you think we would have been violent?" And I said, "Yeah. Oh, yeah. I thought you would have been violent. I saw it in this house. I saw you hit Mom. I saw you beat her. You know—yeah, and I saw how you beat kids" [at the school where he taught]—this was—you know, he'd be in jail today for what he did to kids in school. You know, throw them up against the locker, you know, that kind of stuff. He was the big football coach, right? And, uh, Dad said, "I don't like the word 'gay.'" I said, "I don't care if you don't like it. That's the term we use." And, so, we did not communicate at all for a year. Nothing at all between us. Um [My mother] stayed at the apartment when I was at work and talking to Ben, because she blamed him for me being gay, it was "all his fault." [According to her,] I wouldn't be gay if it hadn't been for Ben. And so—And so, I never heard from them, and I never contacted them until the day Ben died, and my brother called my parents and said, um, "I don't care what you think of your son, about whether he's a gay man or not, but someone he loves very much is dying, and you call him." So, I got home from the hospital. It was, like, 1:00 in the morning, uh, and there was a message on the answering—we had the answering machine. There was a message on the answering machine. It was my mom and dad, and in my father's voice, I could hear it. If he could have turned back time, if he could have done anything to make it better, he would have done it. You know, he was so remorseful and felt so guilty about the way he had treated me and the way he had treated Ben. You know, it was really, really heartfelt, and I could just—I felt it, and I really felt it here. My mother, not so much. So, after Ben died, there was a sort of slow reconciliation process, um, that happened, and we'd have conversations about the weather, you know.

Many gay men, including me, seem to find love and support, understanding, and lack of judgment from their brothers. When I came out to my family, my brother Tony was fully present and supportive. This love and support, clear in Tom's story, was similar for Lorenzo and his two brothers, "And I told my brother. And he's like, 'Yeah, I kinda always knew.' And then, I told my other brother and, um, I knew they wouldn't react negatively to it."

Unlike Tom or Lorenzo, the reactions of his family when Juan came out were full of the familiar chaos, concern, and confusion but ultimately love. Juan felt compelled to speak his truth to his parents in part due to a nationally known crisis—the Pulse Nightclub shooting. Similar to Yasar, alcohol played a role, and he didn't plan out his disclosure:

So I was hung over from that [drinking the night before] and so I was feeling like— it was like the Orlando shooting and me liking this guy, and also the alcohol, that there was one day when I was just really, really, really depressed. And, obviously, it was because I was under the influence, too, but I was contemplating suicide, um. I just walked around the street thinking about it. Like how should I do it? Like, when and like I—I got on—on a bridge and I was like really, really considering it. And I was like, "You know what? I have to tell my parents. If they disown me, that's—that's still going to be a weight off my shoulders, you know, like, if they disown me, at least I'll know that that's what they did." Whereas, now I was living this—like what are they going to do? Are they still going to love me? Like are they—is their love really unconditional, I guess? I got back home and I was crying and I was contemplating if I should call them. But then actually my dad Face-timed me and then he, um, asked me how everything was. But I was—I was like trying to pull off a normal conversation but then I started crying. And then he asked if everything was okay and I just started crying more. And then he said, "Um, you don't have to tell me. I think I know." And then I had like a mini heart attack and I started crying more because I had no idea that—obviously like he's your parent, so—but like in my mind he had no idea. So then he starts crying, too, and he's like—like, "It's okay. We—you are who you are and it's going to take us a while to accept, but, um, don't—don't sweat it too much." And then my mom actually had no idea just because gay isn't really a thing in—being gay isn't really a thing in China. So, she was just like—I think she was in shock. She didn't say much, but she was like, "It's okay. It's okay." She was like, "It's okay. Like don't cry." But like [Dad's] like, "I think I know." As in, "I think I know what you're going to say." Because I was like, "I don't—I can't say it." And he was like, "I think I know what you're going to say." And, um so later he told me that he knew, but my—my mom sincerely didn't have an idea. But, uh so I wasn't with them after I came out, but my sister was with them and she told me they didn't sleep for four days and they were just crying all night. But like to me they—they were very calm and they really gathered themselves. Yeah, and my sister said that they were—they like lost it. Like, when—when they weren't talking to me. But yeah, they seem okay with it. Um, no—they are okay with it, but I can tell it still makes them really uncomfortable.

Fearing similar negative reactions from his parents, Huang suppressed his sexuality in high school and only emerged as a gay man after he left his family home and started college. Huang eloquently depicted the context of his nurturing yet very strict and demanding Chinese home as follows:

I was the oldest of two and, even my father was not born here. He was born in Hong Kong and it was a very strict upbringing. You know, when my parents got together, they met here in the US, but were poor. We didn't have a whole lot. My dad was really a hard-working guy, very, very blue-collar. Worked at the restaurants for a long—his entire life, basically. And there was a lot of expectations that, you know, I would take care of the family and all that. And it was very strict. We had to eat, you know, at a certain time. We had to do things a certain way. A lot of traditions, was very traditional. I mean, I got punished if I didn't [do] the multiplication times-table correct. You know, I had to get A's. I had to get A's, there was no such thing as a B. . . . We didn't have any money. . . . And the only way we could get out of it is via education. [Growing up and marrying a Chinese woman] was implicit and explicit; we went to church every Sunday. And I was an altar boy. And so, even with the Catholic church, you know, it's very much—And I went to an all-boys Catholic high school, was the expectation was to—you know, the notion of a same-sex marriage back then did not even exist. And even in 1992 . . . People were dying of AIDS as well.

Given his home life, Huang patiently waited to fulfill his sexual desires and realize his sexual identity. It was only his husband Walter's death that predisposed him to disclose his identity to his parents:

Walter was the one. He's the soul mate. And he and I got together. We lived together. And for the first couple of years that we were living together, my parents only knew him as a roommate. And he always came to all the family functions. He actually was the one who married my sister-in-law and my brother. He was ordained as a—whatever, a Universal Life church, minister. And um, he passed away, suddenly. And when he passed away, my parents—my mom actually said the words that, "Oh, he's an angel. He's an angel now, watching over you, and you'll—watching over all of us." And I broke down and said, "You know, he's not only an angel, he was my husband. He was the one who took care of me. He was my life partner." [. . .] And I actually said it. I felt like I had to say it, to give him the credit. And, um, it's when she finally broke down and my dad was there too, and the two of them were like, and she was like, "You don't have to say it. You don't have to say it out loud. It's not like we didn't know."

FORCED OUT TO PARENTS

Jim, a member of the Stonewall Generation, didn't have the opportunity to tell his parents, neither by choice nor by the result of a crisis, before they found out on their own.

He ended up in this less than ideal situation when his parents inadvertently found out at that he was gay when he was 22 through a letter he had received from his partner Joseph. After completing his undergraduate studies, Jim began teaching high school English and drama classes, all the while engaged in a long-distance relationship with his lifelong partner Joseph. Upon finding the letter between their son and his partner, Jim's parents reacted strongly:

They found the letter, and I did not back down. And my mother was hysterical, in tears. My father was very, very angry. And um I couldn't lie to them. And I kept saying, "It doesn't change my relationship with you. I still love you. You should still love me. But this is reality. This is how I feel. And I'm not saying it's going to be

forever. This is the way it is right now." [My parents said] "Well, we've got to get
you into therapy. We've got to get you into . . . we've got to fix you. We've got to
fix you." And she was—my mother was beyond words without—the boundaries
were crossed in terms of her with me, big time. I mean, I don't even know how to
use the words, but she was lying on the floor, hysterically crying. So I finally went to
bed that night, and I was starting to think, "What the hell am I doing here? This
can't go away." I actually felt up to that point, that if I ever did anything that was
outside the world of the family: marrying a Black girl, uh anything that would go
against—it would be not accepted, and it would be very, very, very hard for them
to live with it. They were more concerned about the relatives, they were very con-
cerned about the neighbors, they were concerned about every—my future. And um
I didn't back down.

After countless arguments, it was obvious that the difficulties at home
would never subside. Though Jim went to a therapist for a short time, he
actually helped Jim grapple with and accept his identity—not "repair him,"
as his mother had hoped, only exacerbating the situation. Jim knew it was
time to move out:

It was not a good situation. So Joseph would come up on weekends, and I started
looking for an apartment. And I found an apartment in a very bad neighborhood—
the only apartment I could afford. My starting salary at teaching was $7,500.

Despite the advances that have been made, this type of "forced outing"
and parental reaction still occurs for some LGBTQ people. Four decades
later, Miguel's story of coming out to his mother didn't differ in its essence
from that of Jim's in the 1970s. Recall that Miguel was raised by parents of
Guatemalan ancestry; his coming out was forced, like Jim's, but in this case
due to photographs of him and his boyfriend at the time, Roland:

I think mutual friends of ours had taken some pictures of us at a, at, like, a party,
or, like, we were outside at the arboretum or something in Boston. And I was given
the camera. I went to go develop the pictures myself. I went to go pick them up—or
I wanted to—but my mother had already picked them up for me because they were
under my last name. She picked up the pictures. She saw what was on the camera,
and she immediately started, like, flipping out at me. It was a picture of me and my
boyfriend at the time, like, holding each other, like hugging each other. And so she
saw the pictures. She threw it at me. She, like, started screaming, started being re-
ally, like, tormented because, you know, she couldn't fathom that her son was gay.
But she didn't tell anybody. It wasn't until I told my sister later on and that's when
my sister also flipped out—was not accepting of it at all. And then [I told my mom
I was gay the next day]. I was, like, freaked out. My mom was just totally freaked

out. So I told my sister. My sister was not cool with it either, and we started to fight. It got physical. She slapped me across the face. I started trying to choke her out. We, like, we were really violent with each other. And then, I, like, ran out of the house, and I was just like, I'm done. I basically came back that night, um, to see if it would be okay, like, safe to go back home. And my mother was, like, not happy with me. My sister had told her what had happened about what I had said to her, and the fight then ensued afterward, and she was, she's like, I don't want you in this house. So I had to leave. I grabbed a bag. Filled it with as much clothes as possible. It was around, like, 8:00, 9:00 at night probably. Like, so it was already dark out. It was, like, around my senior year of high school. I was, like, 16, 17 years old. And I, I took the bus, or, and the train all the way to my boyfriend's house in the south end of Boston. He lived in these projects building called the Cathedrals. They were for projects. And, um, yeah, the rest of the night's kind of a blur. But at—for the most part, his mother understood why I was there.

After coming out to his brothers, Lorenzo disclosed his identity to his mother but not his father, who only learned about his son's sexuality through reading his journal:

We [my mother and I] were just in the house. And I remember, I said, "I gotta talk to you." And I started telling her and, of course, I started blubbering for no apparent reason. I don't know why I was crying, but I did. And so, she starts crying because I'm crying. And then, I tell her. I said, "I'm gay." She's like, "No, no, no. This can't be." I was like, "Mom, please." I said, "You know it's true." And, so she said, "I kinda did, and I just didn't—I really hoped that it was just, you know, a passing thing." She goes, "Don't tell your father. It's gonna be very bad." Because she was—was keeping—literally, my Mother would do anything to keep everything on the status quo, made—forcing me to play basketball and go to basketball camp, which I hated basketball. I hated it. But, "Go, please, you'll keep the peace." "Okay." So, I—here I am, 14 years old, being shipped off to play basketball with other boys from my town which clearly knew—or their sixth sense was operating and mine wasn't because I—either that, or I thought I was much better at hiding my sexuality than I was—not—probably not really. They all knew. Um, it was kinda rough, um, that telling—telling the people that were closest to me at that moment. Um, I did not ever, actually, tell my dad.

Despite never having any formal communications, when Lorenzo's father found and read Lorenzo's journal, his response was just as bad as both Lorenzo and his mother expected:

Oh, he went ballistic. He came up to my room, slammed the door. My dad's a big outdoorsman; I liked it, too. I was raised with hunting and fishing and doing all that stuff, like camping. . . . So I had a gun in my room. I mean, not a pistol.

I had a rifle in my room. It was mine. And he just was pissed, and he picked it up, and he was marching up and down my room, and I'm like looking; I'm like sliding up on my nightstand, looking for the bullets. I'm like, "I didn't leave them in there, did I?" And I know I didn't. I was like, "Phew!" in my mind, going, "Thank god I didn't." Because he was so enraged that I was gay. [He was screaming] "Yeah, you're a faggot? You wanna suck somebody's dick? Uh, this is bullshit. You gotta get out of this fucking house. You gotta get out." He was—and it like—as he's talking, I'm like, "Okay." I was like, "Fine." I was hurt, but what was I going to do? Fight him? I went to the bar that night. And I'm sitting at the bar, and it came up, and they said, "Well, why do you have a backpack with you?" And I told them, and they were—all the guys who had come out already were like, "Oh, honey. Don't worry," and, you know–I, yeah—I was crying. They were crying. And my friend, Jack, happened to—his roommate happened to be away. They just got a new house. They were looking for a third roommate.

And while Lorenzo's father owned a gay bar, and may have himself experimented in same-sex behaviors, he sought to cure his son:

Well, when I was 21, he decided he was going to send me to a psychiatrist, to get fixed. Yeah. I'm gonna get fixed by Dr. M . . . and I was sitting there by myself, for a few minutes. And it was a Saturday morning. And I heard them—I'm going to use the term "her"—come in. Heard her come in. Because there was not an ounce of masculinity to that man, at all. And he came in with his coffee, his Sergio Valenti sweat suit, and all his baubles on. "Hi, how are you? So, we're gonna talk about"—like, "Are you joking? You're gonna fix me?" I was like, "Sweet"—I was like, "Sweetheart, you're gayer than I am." You know? And whatever he did—apparently, this guy fixed his friend's son. Who that friend's son is, I don't know. I went to him twice, in which he ultimately, apparently, decided to tell everything to my father that I said in the sessions—which is a huge breach of ethics, as you know. But—and I didn't know that at the time, my father and I were having an argument a couple years later, like a brawl, like a screaming brawl—all-out brawl. My father said, "Oh, and Dr. M tells me you think I'm gay." I'm like, "Oh." Like, "Oopsie." Uh, I was a little stunned by that. I'm like, "Okay, I can't fight back now."

UNSPOKEN TELLING

Like Lorenzo and his father, some gay men never utter the words "I am gay" to their parents. Instead, an unspoken understanding develops over time. This unspoken understanding is how my husband Bobby conveyed his sexuality to his parents—there was never a direct discussion nor conversation. As my colleague Michael LaSalla indicates,[3] coming out is critical for the well being of gay couples, and so when Bobby and I were married he invited his father to our wedding. Thus, he did eventually come out. Though somewhat more common for members of the AIDS and Stonewall generations, this approach to nonverbal disclosure seems to have mostly fallen out of favor among men of the Queer Generation.

For 62-year-old Ryan, the process of coming out to his parents happened naturally and nonverbally, despite the fact that he came of age as a gay man prior to the Stonewall Riots. Unlike many of these stories, there was no critical moment of disclosure that occurred, a situation that may ultimately undermine one's self-esteem. Rather there was an understanding and limited discussion, likely shaped by his Irish American heritage. His work as a drag entertainer in his early 20s probably tipped them off as well:

> I really didn't have to come out to my family. They knew. They knew. I was [a] screaming queen. Mary, I was—I was—I was a screaming queen. They knew. Well, I was in my 20s—early 20s—when I started doing drag, dad knew that I was doing drag and he said you can't go out of the house in drag. I started drag in a little—a little bar in Newark, New Jersey. Okay, he knew because people [knew]. He knew I was—he knew I was doing drag and he knew I was—and he knew I was gay. He knew since I was a kid. They both knew. My mom—I remember living—I was on Broadway—living on Broadway in Newark, New Jersey, and I was 15 and my mom was watching—was watching the television or listening to the radio and Stonewall was going on. I remember her coming in and saying, "Your friends are acting up in New York City." What more can you say?

Ryan viewed his official coming out to his parents, though he still never openly stated the words, as having taken place in his 30s:

> So mom and dad came to see Don't Tell Mama's [a club in New York City] because my brother has come to see me, my sister has come to see me, and they said why don't you go see him perform? He's really good. So, they finally came and it was wonderful because I—it was the first night—it was the first week. And he [my dad] said, "I loved the show. Well," he said, "You've always—I knew you were funny. You've always been funny." He said, "And your timing is impeccable, but then again, it always was." And I said, "How's that?" He says, "Well, Ryan, you were born to the minute."

For Ryan, it was clear that this event was one with which he felt little emotional connection, speaking in more generic terms about the results of this interaction:

> It was wonderful because as I got older, you're able to talk with your parents more. You know, sometimes you hate your parents or you hate things that they make you

do or they don't let you do or they—when you get older, you start to realize they were doing certain things because 1 because it was their rules and number 2 because they were trying to protect you.

Even with this nonverbal recognition, like many other gay men's parents and families, Ryan's had to realign their relationship with him, and in the process, learn and emerge as parents of a gay child. Ryan experienced this growth in both himself and his father:

Because they knew I was gay, they knew I was carrying on with guys and uh I started doing—and I was going to bars, and then I was performing, and I performed in Bermuda and so—but, my dad—my dad grew in the same way that I did . . . because I was learning [about my gay identity too]: I didn't have [, nor did my parents have,] TV shows [about LGBTQ people] and—and plus, I didn't have drag stars to watch [like] RuPaul.

Stephanos, of the AIDS Generation, also came out to his Polish mother and Greek father nonverbally, seeing this lack of discussion and verbal disclosure as inherent in his culture. He used the term "American" in the following passage—one used by many immigrant families, including my own, to differentiate us from the traditions and ways of Anglo Saxon Americans:

So, obviously he knew, and we never really talked about it, so that was kind of weird that's popped up because he died last year. But it was like I remember thinking that's odd, but he and I never really spoke about much. Personal stuff, like we didn't really have, like that was just not [our family culture]. For some, American families understand that—like always. Like we just didn't talk about those things. Like, and—and by the same token I talked to my sisters since then and they even said when it comes to like—you know they weren't the people that you talk to you about sex or relationships. They weren't very emotive about that, nor do they really wanna to talk about it, and my father I never talked to about it.

It also appears that Stephanos sought his independence as a way to avoid this conservation about his sexual identity:

And I think we tried to talk about it a couple times but she'd [my mom would avoid it] . . . . At that point I was like I was also financially independent. I was like I got a school scholarship and everything, and I didn't really rely on them. My whole thing was I always worked a lot because I didn't want [to depend on them]. I always figured you know like strings with any money you took from my parents, so I never wanted anything from them. So, I was kind of financially independent, and then that in a lot of ways enabled me to be like—I just don't really care to talk about it with them.

Stephanos immersed himself in his education and schooling, returning home to upstate New York during the summers, when he would work at the local gay club. Aside from directly coming out to his parents, he seemed to be actualized as a gay man in every other way:

Oh, I didn't talk to my [parents about being gay]—and actually I wouldn't. Once I got to that one year and I like read everything I can—by the time I got to college I mean I was like really gay. Like, I was like super, like Mr. Gay, like I'm like proud to be gay. I tried to talk about it to my mother once. She'd cry, I just dropped it.

Even if Stephanos tried communicating with his parents, there seems to have been no cognitive or emotional space for such a conversation. He was met with the same resistance from his parents as Jim, although with much less communication and discussion about his sexuality took place. In the end, though, he seems fine with that knowledge and continues to live his life openly, even if he doesn't discuss it directly with his family.

Similarly, Jason, age 67, never verbally came out to his parents. He took steps to avoid any possibility of such conversations with either parent, but specifically with his mother, with whom he regularly spent time with after his parents divorced in the early 1980s. He knew his mother had denial issues when it came to any challenging situations or emotions, so he decided to take a more compartmentalization approach, keeping his sexual identity separate from other aspects of his life, especially when it came to his family.

She [my mother] couldn't conceive of [divorce] because she was an old Greek lady. You know, she went through all this stuff—denying, denying, boxing things—so that she could keep that [the illusion of her marriage] alive. What I learned from them [my parents] is keeping things in boxes and filing them away to keep the hurt away. Um, so, the bullying I had in junior high and stuff like that—I pushed that away, and, uh, I put [it] in the box, and—pfft! Next! Because you've got to survive, and that's what my mother did.

Jason's life narrative and inability to be open with his family provides insight into much of who he is today—a gay man defined greatly by his physical appearance, sexual proclivity, and sexual behavior. The Jason portrayed during this interview is in part explained by the compartmentalization modeled by his mother's life and marriage, and his decision to hide his gay identity from her. It is rooted in hiding and denial. And during this interview it was clear that Jason was hiding even from us in the same way he hid who he was from his mother. It is likely that this lack of disclosure has led to a limited integration of his gay identity with other aspects of his very full and rich life, and in the absence of such integration, his gay identity is tied firmly and solely to his sexual exploits. Perhaps the self that Jason portrays would have been different had Jason lived openly and honestly with his family. Instead, the Jason we see wears a mask at all times likely in fear that the true Jason would not be loved.

However, it has been debated whether it is essential for all gay men to verbally disclose their status in an effort to fully find themselves and self-actualize. In the cases of Ryan and Stephanos, both men seem to live proud lives as gay men, without ever having had to come out to their parents. Conscious of the fact that there are varying dynamics in different cultures, verbal discourse may not be the only path for fulfillment as a gay man, and espousing such a notion would be rooted in a white cisgender privileged perspective.

I turn again to my Rutgers colleague Michael LaSalla, a social worker who has conducted extensive research on coming out, explained that though there may be some benefits for gay men who verbally disclose their sexual identity to their parents, and in turn receive their support, he was reluctant to flat-out state that direct disclosure is essential to mental health or self-actualization. In fact, his research and clinical experience suggested that many Latino and Asian families deal with the situation nonverbally. He also mentioned how several gay men he had worked with over the years had pushed the issue and came out directly, only to be told by parents that they had basically known, but "Why did you have to tell us?" By avoiding the conversation all together, these families felt they could maintain connections and skirt any conflict related to the parent's personal, cultural, or religious objections to their sons' gay identity. Of course the issue then becomes, how do men within these families manage their mental health and ability to be comfortable with their gay identity without coming out to their parents?

A recent analysis of data from the 2002 Behavioral Risk Factor Surveillance System in Massachusetts found[15] that across generations, gay men who do not come out to their parents do not experience any higher negative health consequences such as binge drinking, illicit drug use, cigarette smoking, and elevated mental health problems. However among those who had disclosed their identities, gay and bisexual men with unsupportive parents indicated higher lifetime drug use and depression. Meanwhile, coming out to parents who end up being supportive has the most beneficial impacts on mental health.[16] Such findings suggest that disclosure of sexual identity must be considered in light of potential parental reaction, which can be wide and varied, especially when coming out to fathers,[17] ranging from acceptance and support to physical violence.[18-21]

In effect one size doesn't fit all: individuals must weigh the pros and cons. For some, nondisclosure may ultimately be the best option. For example, research supports that careful consideration should be given to coming out to parents who hold strong religious beliefs, conservative political views, and rigidity in thinking.[18] While initial reactions range drastically, it is also imperative to note that parental attitudes and reactions have been found to change over time as their love of their children wins out over their preconceived notions.[22] Unfortunately, there is no certainty that such an evolution will occur in my lifetime.

FINAL THOUGHTS

As shown through these stories, negative family reactions to identity disclosure are not confined to the older generations alone. Nor are the stories of acceptance and love confined solely to younger men. Coming out was not uniformly challenging and devastating for the men of the Stonewall and AIDS generations or uniformly calm for the men of the Queer Generation. These parental reactions—whether to direct disclosure, forced conversations or outing, or nonverbal understanding—can be vastly different, even within each generation. All of these individual experiences are shaped by the attachment of the parents with their child, the family's culture, and ultimately the ability for a child and their parents to effectively realign their relationships in light of their new reality.

These coming out experiences, especially in relation to our parents and families, shadow so much of our lives, rooted in the feeling of difference that precedes our abilities to understand our sexuality. So while "blowing over" may symbolically be the metaphor used by Jeremy when explaining how his parents reacted to his disclosure, the fact is that for all of us there is an ongoing challenge to negotiate our sexuality throughout our lives. Even after our families know who we are, we continue to seek integration of our sexual identity with all other aspects of our being, an enduring effort shaped by feelings of otherness deeply embedded in our emotional lives.

REFERENCES

1. Cohen KM, Savin-Williams RC. Developmental perspectives on coming out to self and others. *The lives of lesbians, gays, and bisexuals: Children to adults.* Orlando, FL: Harcourt Brace College Publishers; 1996:113–151.

2. Savin-Williams RC. Coming out to parents and self-esteem among gay and lesbian youths. *J Homosex.* 1989;18(1–2):1–35.

3. LaSala MC. Gay male couples: the importance of coming out and being out to parents. *J Homosex.* 2000;39(2):47–71.

4. Perrin-Wallqvist R, Lindblom J. Coming out as gay: a phenomenological study about adolescents disclosing their homosexuality to their parents. *Soc Behav Pers.* 2015;43(3):467–480.

5. McDonald GJ. Individual differences in the coming out process for gay men: implications for theoretical models. *J Homosex.* 1982;8(1):47–60.

6. Grafsky EL, Hickey K, Nguyen HN, Wall JD. Youth disclosure of sexual orientation to siblings and extended family. *Fam Relat.* 2018;67(1):147–160.

7. Sullivan M, Wodarski JS. Social alienation in gay youth. *J Hum Behav Soc Environ.* 2002;5(1):1–17.

8. Willoughby BL, Doty ND, Malik NM. Parental reactions to their child's sexual orientation disclosure: a family stress perspective. *Parent Sci Pract.* 2008;8(1):70–91.

9. LaSala MC. Lesbians, gay men, and their parents: family therapy for the coming-out crisis. *Fam Process.* 2000;39(1):67–81.

10. Savin-Williams RC, Dube EM. Parental reactions to their child's disclosure of a gay/lesbian identity. *Fam Relat.* 1998:47(1):7–13.

11. Ben-Ari A. The discovery that an offspring is gay: parents', gay men's, and lesbians' perspectives. *J Homosex.* 1995;30(1):89–112.

12. Grov C, Bimbi DS, Nanin JE, Parsons JT. Race, ethnicity, gender, and generational factors associated with the coming-out process among lesbian, and bisexual individuals. *J Sex Res.* 2006;43(2):115–121.

13. Boxer A, Cook J, Herdt G. To tell or not to tell: patterns of self-disclosure to mothers and fathers reported by gay and lesbian youth. In: Pillemer K, McCartney K, eds. *Parent–child relations across the lifespan.* New York: Oxford University Press;1991:59–93.

14. Gao G. *Most Americans now say learning their child is gay wouldn't upset them.* Washington, DC: Pew Research Center; 2015.

15. Rothman EF, Sullivan M, Keyes S, Boehmer U. Parents' supportive reactions to sexual orientation disclosure associated with better health: results from a population-based survey of LGB adults in Massachusetts. *J Homosex.* 2012;59(2):186–200.

16. Ryan C, Huebner D, Diaz RM, Sanchez J. Family rejection as a predictor of negative health outcomes in white and Latino lesbian, gay, and bisexual young adults. *Pediatrics.* 2009;123(1):346–352.

17. Jadwin-Cakmak LA, Pingel ES, Harper GW, Bauermeister JA. Coming out to dad: young gay and bisexual men's experiences disclosing same-sex attraction to their fathers. *Am J Mens Health.* 2015;9(4):274–288.

18. Baiocco R, Fontanesi L, Santamaria F, et al. Negative parental responses to coming out and family functioning in a sample of lesbian and gay young adults. *J Child Fam Stud.* 2015;24(5):1490–1500.

19. Daly SC, MacNeela P, Sarma KM. When parents separate and one parent "comes out" as lesbian, gay or bisexual: sons and daughters engage with the tension that occurs when their family unit changes. *PLoS One.* 2015;10(12):e0145491.

20. Livingston J, Fourie E. The experiences and meanings that shape heterosexual fathers' relationships with their gay sons in South Africa. *J Homosex.* 2016;63(12):1630–1659.

21. Willoughby BL, Malik NM, Lindahl KM. Parental reactions to their sons' sexual orientation disclosures: the roles of family cohesion, adaptability, and parenting style. *Psychol Men Masc.* 2006;7(1):14.

22. Samarova V, Shilo G, Diamond GM. Changes in youths' perceived parental acceptance of their sexual minority status over time. *J Res Adolesc.* 2014;24(4):681–688.

CHAPTER 5

Otherness

A s evident throughout the interviews conducted for this book, the challenges of being gay start at a very young age and persist throughout the course of our lives. During that time, we seek to become self-actualized by integrating our gay identity with other aspects of who we are as people, as a whole. These processes are not only complicated by ongoing societal conditions but also exacerbated by the gay community itself, where conceptions of maleness and normalcy, issues of racism, and conditions that facilitate and fuel drug use and risky sex shape so much of our experience. At the center of all these challenges is an embedded feeling of otherness that is only emphasized through the need to come out repeatedly.

Each and every gay man interviewed told stories characterized by language reflecting their feelings of otherness during their childhood and formative years. This sensibility that starts at a young age often permeates much of our lives, as noted by Tom:

> From my first memories on, I knew that I was different. Of course, I didn't know what that difference meant, and as I grew older, I felt more and more isolated because I felt more and more different, and that difference wasn't "other than," it was "less than." So I remember at the age of five, telling my mother that when I grew up, I was never going to get married and that I was moving to New York. I don't know how I knew that, but that's what I told her.

Otherness, that sense that we are different and living on the outside of heteronormative society and culture, is often the way we as gay men understand ourselves, and if unchecked it can serve as a source of loneliness and social isolation, contributing to other psychosocial burdens that diminish our health. It all begins in our youth, as misunderstood young children who cannot conceptualize our feelings in a concrete manner, leading to adolescence and young adulthood, when certain aspects of who we are, specifically our gay identity, start to become clearer.

Even in today's more progressive era, in which imagery and depictions of gay men are more prevalent in mainstream media and entertainment than ever before, and there is a greater widespread acceptance of the lesbian, gay, bisexual, transgender, and queer (LGBTQ) community, an underlying pulse of confusion, judgment, contempt, and hate toward gay men still exists, and at times rears its ugly head, perpetuating this sense of otherness in our lives. Perhaps these experiences are less frequently manifested as macro- than microaggressions; yet as noted in the beginning of the book, microaggressions can be just as powerful and damaging as macroaggressions.

Gay men's relationships to the microsystem of our families and the macrosystem of society, as well as contexts in between such as our neighborhoods or ethnic communities, serve as the source and weight of the otherness we must endure. Coming out to parents serves as an initial step for many as a means to state and own their otherness. Our lifelong trajectory of gay identity development is then the process by which we begin to ultimately make sense and integrate this otherness, diminishing the negative impact that feelings of our "difference" have in our lives. Nonetheless, this outsider status and feeling, this sensibility of otherness, comes to shape the choices and decisions we make, the behaviors we enact, the relationships we develop including seeking out older men, and the type of lives we end up leading.

SOURCES OF OTHERNESS

Gay men's feelings of otherness begin at a young age. The inherent feeling that something is "different" about them, as expressed in many of the men's stories throughout the book, eventually gives way to the understanding that this otherness is an indicator of sexual identity. That feeling of being different never dissipates and is only reinforced by social settings and groups, such as families, neighborhoods, schools, communities, religious congregations, and workplaces, and within local, state, and federal governments. Speaking of the current sociopolitical climate, one of the men interviewed said:

There's still a lot of ignorance out there. There's still a lot of bullying out there. There's still a lot of hate crimes that's happening. But there's still a lot of negativity going on when dealing with gay people. And it's not like people don't know. People do know. But they're not aware of it, just like, you know, AIDS has been out for a long time, and even when I found out that I was positive. I knew about it. I just didn't care about it. I didn't educate myself on it. So you have a lot of gay youth out here that's not educating themselves about it. Because anything can happen. I know a bunch of people that got killed—well, mostly trannies, or drag queens, because they think they can just go out there and try to fool someone, and then the person finds out and then just totally blank out on them and kill them. The same goes for those young gay guys aren't careful. I think that's important.

Such social, emotional, and physical victimization has persisted for decades. Unwarranted violence took the lives of transgender activist Marsha P. Johnson, college student Matthew Shepard, Italian fashion designer Gianni Versace, and countless less visible members of the LGBTQ community, crimes that have gone unsolved in the case of Johnson or under-punished in the case of Shepard. In Versace's case, the mishandling and disregard for the lives of gay men facilitated Andrew Cunanan's killing streak, leading to the execution of the designer in 1997. No amount of *Will & Grace* or *Queer Eye* will improve these conditions, and these circumstances continue to define the lives of gay men, perhaps even being exacerbated with the vitriol of the populist conservative political agenda that has emerged and gained momentum throughout the world in the first 2 decades of the 21st century.

When gay men flip on the news and are hit with this reality or, even worse, experience violence firsthand, it becomes impossible to see ourselves as anything else than "other" or even "disposable." In light of these aggressions toward our community, our feelings of otherness continue to be inflamed, creating wounds even for those of us who are secure in our identities. That's why seemingly small microaggressions, such as the 2017 Supreme Court decision in *Masterpiece Cake Shop vs. Colorado Civil Rights* can still have such a strong effect on LGBTQ people. In this case, a Lakewood, Colorado bakery refused to bake a cake for a same-sex couple, claiming First Amendment rights to refuse the newlyweds. As noted by ACLU's David D. Cole, such an act is equivalent to the bakery seeking "a constitutional right to hang a sign in its shop window proclaiming, "Wedding Cakes for Heterosexuals Only.""[1]

For many heterosexual individuals, such a story may not seem all that abhorrent, but that's in part due to the fact that they too easily understand gay men as "others." Otherness is based on a relational dynamic between two groups. The construct creates an artificial dichotomy between the self and the person, or people, deemed the other. The other is then considered different—a deviation from what is "normal"—particularly if their characteristics are considered strange, odd, exotic, or bizarre.[2] The group in power assigns otherness to those who are unlike them. The main problem with this construction is that it very often involves creating enemies of, or demonizing, the "other." Once the damage is done, it's hard, if not impossible, to reverse. For example, in 2013 the British government pardoned Alan Turing, mentioned in chapter 2, and thousands of other gay men for being gay, thereafter.[3] But in doing so the British government did nothing but perpetuate their otherness. What the government perceived as a positive step forward, ended as a sad reminder to gay men on how we have been harassed, victimized, castrated, and killed, even when we are geniuses, heroes, and patriots like Turing.

Norwegian scholar Thomas Harding succinctly describes[4] the experience of gay men as noted in the language to which they are often exposed, pointing to phrases like "these people" and "that way inclined," statements highly reminiscent of those I heard in my youth by the Greek men with whom I was raised. Such language acts as a source of maintenance of power and exclusion by certain classes of heterosexual men. In his 1994 essay, "Masculinity as Homophobia,"[5] sociologist Michael Kimmel described the otherness perpetuated on gay men as "the politics of exclusion," explaining that many heterosexual men attempt to push gay men to the margins or demean them in an effort to "reground their sense of themselves without those haunting fears and that deep shame that they are unmanly and will be exposed by other men." Simply put, insecurities lead to the creation of an "other." Identifying a person or group as the other makes it easier to accept or perpetuate hateful or degrading acts toward them, especially microaggressions.

There is ample evidence to suggest that gay men and LGBTQ people more broadly experience microaggressions routinely,[6] leading to their marginalization and otherness. Psychologist Kevin Nadal, a fellow New Yorker and gay man, effectively describes microaggressions as "brief and commonplace daily verbal, behavioral, or environmental indignities, whether intentional or unintentional, that communicate hostile, derogatory, or negative slights and insults toward members of oppressed groups."[7] Nadal vividly calls the microaggressions that LGBTQ youth experience "a death by a thousand cuts,"[8] depicting the power that they have in undermining gay men's well-being throughout their lives. These thousand cuts only serve to reinforce otherness, starting at a young age.

Tom, for example, experienced this sense of otherness during his childhood and adolescence as his sexual identity was gestating. Unlike his football-playing brother and football-loving father, the coach of the high school team, Tom was more interested in music, leading to demeaning experiences throughout high school:

> So, it was you know, it was never overt physical. But, you know, something? It's not the physical that is, I think, most hurtful. It's that kind of condemnation, I'll call it, from your peers that is most damaging . . . You know, I played the clarinet. I got straight As. My brother got Bs and Cs. And, so there was this difference, I think, from the beginning, my brother was jealous of me. I didn't realize that that's what it was at the time, but that kind of fueled his anger at me, and he just followed along with his classmates with the kind of taunting and teasing.

Tom's experience of feeling different or being excluded followed him from school to home:

> So, even at the dinner table: I remember that we had dinner at the exact same time, 5:30, every day, and, so the conversation around the dinner table, even I felt excluded from that, because there wasn't anything I felt, uh, that I could bring up and that we would talk about that would be of interest to them.

For Ryan, also a member of the Stonewall Generation, these experiences of difference, and ultimately rejection, took place in the church:

> My father was really great when it came to religious things. My father encouraged us to go to church. Any church we wanted to. My father didn't go to church. My father was a Mason. Mom went to Methodist? Presbyterian? One or the other in Jersey. He encouraged us to go to church. We could go to the church we wanted to and I went to church until I was about 16 years old and I was asked to leave. I was a flamboyant queen and finally one day uh a minister came in and said, "Um, I think it's best that you don't come here anymore."

These feelings of rejection and difference also impacted Ryan's life at high school and were still present even some 30 years after he had graduated:

> I went to the 30-year reunion and there were boys there who were married, had wives. [During high school] they were straight boys, but they wanted a blow job. That didn't make them gay. That just made them horny. So, there were a couple guys and one come on over. And I sat there knowing that I had sucked their dicks and their wives were there. But I also was sad—you had the black kids on one side, you had the white kids on the other side, and the misfits in the middle. High school all over again.

Ryan proceeded to describe little hope in the undoing of a tradition of casting out "others" in our country, whether gay men or people of color:

> *And certain places—it's never gonna change. And that's why you have people doing what they're doing, like Donald Trump because people are always going to hate other people. It sucks. Not as well as I do, but it sucks.*

Lorenzo, of the AIDS generation, also expressed feelings of otherness in how it relates to the potential danger of the current political climate:

> *I was very happy to be a gay man up until November [2016]. I honestly have some, opinions about that. I was never frightened about being a gay man, after I came out. I'm more reluctant to be that guy nowadays. I think a lot of people feel emboldened and empowered by what happened in November, in terms of the election. Two or three of my friends had very negative experiences in the weeks after the election. Um, "Yo, faggot!" You get back in [the closet]. A friend of mine bumped into some-body, on Broadway, as a matter of fact. Just came out of a building, bumped: "Oh, I'm sorry." And the guy had a Trump "Make America Great Again" hat on. Bumped into him and he's like, "Yo, you faggot. Watch where you're walking." It's like, "Seriously?" One kid got smacked upside the head by somebody walking on the street. And I'm like, "It starts." You know, as much as we were emboldened by the previous administration, in being allowed to do what we wanna do and say, "We're right behind you. We got your back," now the opposite is happening.*

THE EFFECT ON COMING OUT

The societal factors that lead to the creation of "others" cause many gay men to be hesitant about coming out. Not only does that difference they've al-ways felt pull at them, but it is continuously propagated by the world around them. If they are unable to embrace this otherness and integrate it with the rest of their life, their self-development will be stunted. For example, both the subtle and obvious forms of bigotry resulting from society's creation of "others" negatively impacted Stephanos' coming out process. He always felt as if he was stuck in some way, confronting an obstacle to becoming his true self:

> *I always remember a line from* My So-Called Life: *"people always ask you about your personality like it's a fixed thing like a toaster." I always remember that line, but yeah you feel that you're very fixed—you can't be yourself.*

Similarly for Huang, afraid that being gay would not only perpetuate the otherness that he felt but could also lead to misery in high school—which he attended in the late 1980s to early 1990s—he remained in the closet. His fears weren't unfounded, having witnessed what had occurred to a friend of his who came out at that time:

> My best friend at the time, I had kind of disassociated myself with him because he came out. I mean, he was all about Madonna. His entire locker was nothing but Madonna, Madonna, Madonna. My locker was right next to him, and I was all Janet Jackson. It was all Rhythm Nation, Control. You know, and so, we have like the dueling battles of the divas, but yet, like . . . I didn't even admit to being gay. And he was really brave. He said, "Fuck it. I'm gonna come out." And he did, and he was bullied. Awfully. Awfully.

Jim also spoke of consciously denying his sexuality in the hopes of achieving some sense of "normalcy," despite having a sense of his otherness from a young age:

> I craved a kind of "I am normal," and I never felt normal. Never. Never. Never. And I remember, in sixth grade, being attracted to some boys, which you know, I harbored those feelings. That was not anything that I can [could] discuss. And I remember imagining standing next to a particularly attractive boy at the urinal. And I went, "Oh, my God." And push all that aside. Pushing all that aside, and I remember going shopping, and having boys look at me when I was shopping um in high school. I went, "Oh, my God, these people are looking at me. I guess they want me. But I don't—I'm not—I'm not gay. I'm not gay. I'm not gay."

Many gay men live in this space, riddled with anxiety, scared that their sexuality will diminish or compromise their well-being. For Yasar, this sense of otherness caused him to feel bad about himself, resulting in a need to hide who he was, even at a young age:

> I didn't know any gay people at the time but I knew what it was and I knew what it meant and I could connect it. I was like oh I'm gay but I'm not going to tell anybody or anything, at 7.

So too, Juan describes the experience of otherness, extending his understanding of feeling different to incorporate his race and culture, in addition to his sexual orientation. His words speak to the plight of the Queer Generation today in regard to diversity, intersectionality, and an understanding of self:

> In Mexico I always say they—they assume I'm Chinese. But when I'm in China, they—they sense that there's like—I'm not fully Chinese, but they think I'm

maybe like Filipino or Japanese, so like—and I also lived in Spain and in Spain they—they just assume I'm an immigrant or sometimes they would call me American just because, um, I spoke English. So yeah, it's always been this—this sense of otherness. And then with the gay—like with the aspect of being gay, it's just one more like degree of otherness that it's hard to get used to. I see it as a burden.

For Lorenzo, Jim, and others who are either sent to therapy or forced to "solve their sexuality problem" through religion, feelings of otherness are exacerbated, and in many ways heightened, by overt messaging from parents who portray their children's sexuality as abnormal, bizarre, and morally wrong. Such indignities create havoc in the lives of many young gay men, regardless of when they come of age. This idea was powerfully and painfully shared by Miguel, who used every possible mechanism available to him to cope with his sexual orientation before leaving home:

I continued to smoke weed and find alcohol whenever I could around like 13. I wasn't a heavy drinker, but I used to smoke pot a lot. And, like, smoking weed was sort of, like, an ease out of—it was like a self-medicating thing. Just to drown out everything that happened. Everything. The trauma that was associated with being gay, the—I just didn't want to think about those things anymore. I didn't want to think about being picked on that day. I didn't want to think about not fitting in that day or not having any friends. I didn't want to think about anything. So I just wanted to zone out. So I did that every night on, like, my parents' rooftop. I just, like, snuck out the window, smoked weed, crawled back into bed, prayed for a better day tomorrow.

OTHERNESS AND LONELINESS

There is an inherent sense of sadness and loneliness in Miguel's words. Unfortunately, such experiences are common among those gay men who suffer from loneliness—an epidemic that likely finds its origins in the otherness encountered at a young age. Sociologist Eric Klinenberg notes that the use of the word "epidemic" to describe the phenomenon of loneliness in society is a misnomer,[9] but there is a nuance missing here when it comes to gay men. The notion that loneliness is due simply to social disconnection—isolating oneself—fails to address the conditions that marginalized individuals, such as members of the LGBTQ community, experience when they are overtly as well as subtly shunned.

Loneliness is a palpable reality for gay men—a state that often drives risk and diminishes overall physical and mental health. Journalist Michael

Hobbes articulated the impact of loneliness in the lives of gay men, connecting this burden to feelings of otherness and the masking of sexual identity, in a 2016 article: "Whether we recognize it or not our bodies bring the closet with us into adulthood."[10] This statement perfectly captures the fight against otherness that haunts gay men from a young age.

Social disconnection may be synonymous with loneliness for cisgender white heterosexual men, but for those who do not fit squarely into this bucket of privilege, feelings of otherness perpetuated by society and political leaders fuel loneliness. So while simply "being lonely," a feeling everyone has at times, may not be an epidemic per se, loneliness and the resulting health disparities gay men and other marginalized groups experience—including high rates of substance use and abuse and the associated risk behaviors—are, in fact, epidemic.[11,12]

The desire to feel less alienated also plays a role in many young men's decision to come out to their parents.[13] Still, the underlying loneliness doesn't truly ever go away and continues to permeate their existence, even when they are not physically, romantically, or emotionally alone and even if they have surrounded themselves with caring friends. Tom regularly witnesses this reality in his social work practice:

> A lot of my male gay patients say to me, "You know, uh, I don't have any friends. I don't have any friends." And, so, I talk to them about, "How many friends do you have?" And, they'll start counting, and they'll get up to four, five. I said, "That's great. That's a lot of friends. You may have 5,000 Facebook friends, but those [four or five] are [real] friends."

For Ryan, growing up in a blue-collar neighborhood in northern New Jersey in the 1950s and 1960s, loneliness almost became his mantra, perhaps as means of emphasizing the pain in his life:

> I had no role model, thank you. I had no role model. I had no role model. All my life has been me. I couldn't hide. I've never hid.

Seth, too, understood that his feelings stemmed from a lack of appropriate role models:

> All of our models have been heteronormative. They're, like, how do we, how do we fit, like, into that framework when all we're trying to do is discover who we are. And often finding that when we gravitate to what we know, which is this heteronormative model and see one, on one hand that the heteronormative model is actually broken, and then find ourselves narrowing our scope of being into that

framework, and only to discover that for most people, that's not even—it's not possible.

Feeling "different" or "less than," or "knowing but hiding," leads to ongoing attempts to try to "fit in" and "suffer in silence." Across generations, men suggest that this struggle is not always obvious to their parents, families, and friends. As Tom mentioned:

My father—I always assumed—because we never talked about feelings, we were not a physical family, how's that for stereotype that he didn't approve of me or like me very much, and that was another thing that made me feel, you know, alone. It made me feel alone in my family.

Stephanos felt similar, but in a different era and with a different group of people—his college classmates:

I was kinda fooling around with a friend of mine who was on the crew team. But, that like again, was mostly like mutual masturbation kind of stuff. And, he had a girlfriend, and then it was just—it got weirder and weirder the longer I was there because I realize that if I came out it was—I look like a weirdo if I came out there, so I got really depressed at one point about that because I feel—like by the time of my sophomore year, I was like now if I just come out, I'm just going to be like a weirdo because there's no reason for me not to come out before in this place. Does that make sense?

Yasar's negative emotions associated with his sexuality also led to loneliness and depression, both of which he sought to mask with unhealthy behavior:

I was going through like a depression. Well actually no not yet. But anyways, I was drinking a little bit much around that time because I was still figuring out my sexuality.

As gay men, especially young gay men, attempt to figure out their sexuality, this burden of otherness not only leads to depression, risky sexual behavior, drug use, and diminished health but also to a positive search for role models, for people who may understand what they're going through, or who have gone through these experiences themselves. This search is essentially an effort to understand how to be, and how to cope with being, a gay man, which may result in the development of relationships with older members of the gay community.

When the British series *Queer as Folk* was produced for American television, the character of 15-year-old Nathan, who begins a sexual relationship with Stuart, much his senior, was sanitized so that he became the 17-going-on-18-year-old (i.e., legal) Justin, who strikes up a relationship with a 20-something named Brian. Maybe this change in Justin's age speaks to American attitudes on the subject, but the reality is that many young gay men across generations have found, and continue to find, growth and support in realizing their sexual identities by engaging in intergenerational love. In fact, when the 2017 film *Call Me by Your Name* was released, the actors Armie Hammer and Timothée Chalamet were confronted about the age gap in this love story to which Chalamet responded, "when you see the film and read the book it is so not part of the equation. That's a conversation worth having after people have seen the film. But everyone in my experience who has seen it hasn't had that conversation. Because the relationship couldn't be more consensual and full of love."[14] And it is that love at the center of the relationship that morphs this intergenerational relationship from an act of victimization to an act of empathy, camaraderie, and respect. This idea of love as absolution must be approached with caution.

For young gay men, intergenerational love provides a way for them to grow and learn about themselves as gay men, finding support from an individual or community that helps them chisel away at their feelings of otherness. In the absence of parents who can teach us about how to love another man, let alone have sex with another man, and in light of sex education that fails to include instruction about same-sex intercourse, such relationships are not only logical, but also helpful as we develop in our lives. The uncertainty and alienation that accompanies otherness tends to lessen as we find that we are in fact not alone, that there are many "others" out there, just like us, wrestling the realities of being a gay man at any given time, no matter the social standards or politics of the day.

That said, just like some heterosexual men and women, there are some gay men who take advantage of younger people when they are in a vulnerable state. Predatory or nonconsensual sexual advances are obviously inappropriate, unhelpful, coercive, and criminal and shouldn't be treated glibly. We certainly have come to understand these specific types of sexual experiences of young boys with older men as abuse, especially in light of the behavior of public personas, such as actor Kevin Spacey, who weaponized his coming out as means for trying to excuse his sexual abuse of boys. Reflecting on this idea, a young man who, as a teenager, had been sexually assaulted by conductor James Levine for years described his thoughts in an article that appeared in the *New York Post*:[15]

"I began seeing a 41-year-old man when I was 15, without really understanding I was really 'seeing' him," the alleged victim, now 48, said in a written statement to

the police department. "It nearly destroyed my family and almost led me to suicide. I felt alone and afraid. He was trying to seduce me. I couldn't see this. Now I can."

Suffice it to say that many young gay men have fallen prey to this crime during a period fraught with feelings of otherness, alienation, and fear brought on by identity confusion and a lack of self-development.

This predatory behavior and attitude is not the norm, but challenges exist in delineating a consensual and loving relationship involving an underage man from one that is forced, coerced, and unwanted. Parsing out love and caring from coercion may be hard. Even when a relationship is "consensual," it may be very difficult for a young man who is confused about who he is, and in a state of vulnerability, to be clear in terms of his thoughts and actions, especially when coupled with the sensations of desire and lust. In effect, acts of intergenerational love that may not seem predatory due to the "heat of the moment," may in fact truly be predatory. At the end of the day, a child is still a child and lust has way of getting in the way of good judgment; adults should know better than to take advantage of that situation, even when they are beautifully depicted as is the case in *Call Me by Your Name*.

The challenge in circumstances involving a man below the age of 18 is that it is not readily clear whether he is emotionally equipped to recognize the actions of an older man as harassment or abuse when the sexual and emotional attraction is present for the younger man. Wilson, now 78, vividly recounted his earliest sexual experiences as a preteenager. Though they were both obviously predatory and abusive, he sees them differently:

When I got a little older—I don't remember what happened, say, by the time I was 10 or 11, if I was home alone and he [an uncle] came to visit, he would ask me to take off my clothes and screw me. I used to cry, only because it hurt me, but I wanted him to be a lover. But whenever he would come back, you know, maybe six or eight months later, I wanted it. And that's why I don't keep it in my mind, because I keep—people say, this is child abuse. I say, no, it wasn't, because I could say I got to the point where he didn't ask me to take my clothes off. By the time I was 12, the minute I saw him, I'd take my clothes off. I mean, if we were home alone.

More often than not, however, stories of sexual adventures with older men during one's adolescence were somewhat normal and desirable in the experiences of the men with whom I spoke for this book, as well as for my previous book. In fact, many friends have also shared similar anecdotes. In this particular historical moment, a rush to judgment of wrongdoing regarding such relationships is the norm, but there are more factors to consider than age alone.

For many of the men with whom I spoke, across generations, having sex with older men during or before adolescence was not viewed as shameful, nor did they demonstrate any remorse, regret, or anger. Though a sense of otherness may have contributed to these relationships, these men began to better understand themselves through these experiences. While it was sometimes challenging for me to hear them describe certain relationships as erotic and a fulfillment of their fantasies, I also could understand. My first same-sex relationship was with a man double my age—a notion that seems anathema and repulsive to me as an older man now.

It was legal: I was 18 and the man, whose name was Jim, was 36 when we first met. When we were together, it felt normal, and I didn't feel like an outsider in the way that I had for so many years. Over time, I have come to understand this relationship as predatory and emotionally abusive, but it also allowed me to emerge into my life as a gay man, albeit under the scrutiny and control of a powerful older man. While my experiences were a far cry from those of Wilson or of Lorenzo, raped by a priest at age 12, they have nonetheless shaped me for a very long time. When Jim died in 1986 from complications of AIDS, I felt free.

My relationship with Jim was no different from that of numerous other young gay men searching to find themselves. Seth, now age 48, recounted his sexual experimentation with older men during his adolescent years, at a time when he also was having sex with men his own age:

> I had had some experimentation with guys my age but it was so innocent and normal and in some ways, developmentally normal, and having already had experiences with older men, I looked at it from a position of being just curious, like, what a difference it is to fuck an older guy or a guy who's, you know, maybe ten years older than me and to, you know, jerk off or whatever with, um, someone who's about my age, was completely different. And of course I preferred older men, I was always looking for the older brother/daddy.

Seth proceeded to share a story that took place when he was 16 years old, one that was still highly erotic for him:

> So I eventually found myself at the Bijou [a movie theater], on 3rd Avenue below 14th Street, and yeah, of course they asked me how old I was but all I had to do was say, yeah, I'm of age and they don't care. I met . . . God I used to remember his name so clearly, and so we played there and in the bathroom there, we took this heavy garbage can, we pushed it against the door so nobody could bother us. And then he said, "Well, just come home with me," and it was right here on Waverly, and, at a certain point he said, "So, my partner's gonna be coming home, and he'll like you." So that was my first three-way, they were probably ten years older than I was, and it was, of course, to the moment, the most erotic experience

I've ever had. We smoked pot and played [listened to] Kitaro—it was one of those, it's like, you know, emblazoned on my mind. You know, immediately fell head over heels with these guys, I sent them this huge bouquet of flowers. I mean, it was just nuts.

Jeremy, now 24, also clearly recounted his experiences during his adolescence with a man almost double his age:

I was still 17 at the time, because it was, like, the end of high school. So I wasn't legal. But this guy was older, and he was a teacher in Long Island. And he was, like, well, you know, we can do . . . he was scared, obviously, to try to, but I guess he liked younger guys. So he came and picked me up. He was probably in his 30s. And he came and picked me up in his Hummer, and took me to Long Island. And giving me booze, and food, and we had sex. And then the next day, he brought me back. But then he disappeared. You know what I mean? Which was fine for me. I mean, I don't know. At the time, I was just like, whatever.

When pressed about whether he thought of the event as child abuse, given that he was a minor at the time, Jeremy said:

No. I didn't feel that. But I met him when I was in college because I went to college in Long Island for the first three years. And he said he lost his job for doing it with somebody else, with another kid.

As gay men, we are separated out as "others" almost from birth—we have no role models, we have no appropriate sex education, and we are, for the most part, raised by straight parents. It's little surprise that many of us turn to our "elder statesmen" to teach us the ways of gay. Intergenerational love is common for same-sex individuals and likely has different meaning and value than it does for heterosexual relationships. Some of these relationships are between underage men and women, which at first glance can be framed as child abuse, and in some cases should be. Many people argue that a teenage boy cannot know better and by the very nature of intergenerational relationships the older man is taking advantage of the situation. In some cases this is likely true, but there are also some in which younger gay men enter these partnerships fully aware of what they may hold.

If undertaken with open heart and open mind, such intergenerational love does not have to be seen as predatory—when it is coerced, it is. Having interviewed thousands of men over the course of the last 20 years, however, it has become apparent that there are circumstances in which these situations are simply about finding acceptance; learning about one's self; loving someone else; and not predatory at all. I do not condone sexual relationships with minors—or any predatory relationship—but intergenerational relationships occur in the LGBTQ community frequently. We must all understand their roots to better grasp the maligned experience of gay men today and in the past.

FINAL THOUGHTS

All gay men experience a feeling of otherness throughout their lives, though it is most pronounced at a young age. Such feelings affect decisions on sexual identity disclosure to families, friends, and classmates, and contribute to depression, anxiety, and loneliness, as well as other psychosocial burdens—including homophobia and hypermasculinity—that drives diminished health. These feelings can also, in part, lead to a search for acceptance and affection from older men, with various results.

Psychosocial conditions prevalent in the gay community create stressors that drive health disparities, resulting in an epidemic. These conditions can lead to the risk behaviors evidenced in the lives of some gay men, including substance use and risky sex, which ultimately take their toll on our health individually and as a population. Evidence also shows that focusing solely on behavior will be insufficient in ameliorating health disparities in gay men. Instead, combination approaches must be taken, marrying biomedical, behavioral, and social structures to combat ongoing health issues. Confronting and handling otherness must be at the center of such multipronged approaches, else only the symptoms are treated without fully addressing the cause.

Gay or straight, it's no easy feat to come to terms with one's self, to fully develop an identity that can be thought of as whole. But for gay men, this quest is all the more treacherous, as we are cast as outsiders from the start. As discussed, sources of otherness don't just come from internal feelings, but from the social, cultural, and political environments of the time. Perhaps these social conditions explain why so many gay men have adopted hegemonic conceptions of masculinity—hypermasculinity to compensate for these exclusionary tactics. In return, however, they have created an exclusion and sense of otherness for gay men who are not buff, hypermasculine White doppelgangers of Thor or Captain American—a discriminatory and exclusionary reality understood with great acumen by men of the Queer Generation.

REFERENCES

1. de Vogue A. Supreme Court hears same-sex marriage cake case. *CNN* 2017.
2. Miller J. Otherness. In: Given LM, ed. *The SAGE encyclopedia of qualitative research methods.* Thousand Oaks, CA: SAGE Publications; 2008:587–589.
3. "Alan Turing law": thousands of gay men to be pardoned. *BBC* 2016.
4. Harding T. The construction of men who are nurses as gay. *J Adv Nurs.* 2007;60(6):636–644.
5. Kimmel MS. Masculinity as homophobia. In: Brod H, Kaufman M, eds. *Theorizing masculinities.* Thousand Oaks, CA: SAGE Publications; 1994:119–141.
6. Nadal KL, Rivera DP, Corpus J, Sue D. Sexual orientation and transgender microaggressions. In: Sue D, ed. *Microaggressions and marginality: Manifestation, dynamics, and impact.* Hoboken, NJ: Wiley; 2010:217–240.
7. Nadal KL. Preventing racial, ethnic, gender, sexual minority, disability, and religious micr oaggressions: recommendations for promoting positive mental health. *Prev Couns Psychol.* 2008;2(1):22–27.
8. Nadal KL, Issa M-A, Leon J, Meterko V, Wideman M, Wong Y. Sexual orientation microaggressions: "death by a thousand cuts" for lesbian, gay, and bisexual youth. *J LGBT Youth.* 2011;8(3):234–259.
9. Klinenberg E. Is loneliness a health epidemic? *New York Times* 2018.
10. Hobbes M. The epidemic of gay loneliness. *Huffington Post* 2017.
11. Halkitis PN, Pollock JA, Pappas MK, et al. Substance use in the MSM population of New York City during the era of HIV/AIDS. *Subst Use Misuse.* 2011;46(2–3):264–273.
12. Woody GE, VanEtten-Lee ML, McKirnan D, et al. Substance use among men who have sex with men: comparison with a national household survey. *J Acquir Immune Defic Syndr.* 2001;27(1):86–90.
13. Perrin-Wallqvist R, Lindblom J. Coming out as gay: a phenomenological study about adolescents disclosing their homosexuality to their parents. *Soc Behav Pers.* 2015;43(3):467–480.
14. Wakeman G. Armie Hammer, Timothée Chalamet defend the age gap between their "Call Me By Your Name" characters. *Metro* 2017.
15. Vincent I, Klein M. Legendary opera conductor molested teen for years: police report. *New York Post* 2017.

CHAPTER 6

(Hyper) Masculinity

The question of what it means to "be a man" is one that many men, no matter their sexual orientation, grapple with throughout their lives. Gay men, however, are stuck in a unique position, reconciling this question with their sexual identities, and in turn, affecting their decisions on disclosure. As gay men, we are raised and "nurtured" in a heterocentrist world, likely by heterosexual parents, and some of us grow up in "traditional" families in which patriarchy and rigid conceptions of masculinity are considered normal.[1] Starting at a young age, these circumstances are embedded in verbal and nonverbal messages and rooted in masculine role socialization.[2,3] As a result, we are exposed to the same circumstances that share and reinforce binary gender norms and hegemonic masculinity as any other boy or man. Anxiety and fear about being viewed as different from this heteronormative masculine standard causes many of us to hide our sexual identities or adapt hypermasculine identities to "compensate" for any diminished sense of worth imposed by society.

While we are young boys, we learn to assert our power over girls, as well as other boys who are seen as "different," creating an anxiety within ourselves given our own sense of otherness. As far back as many of us can remember, this pursuit of dominance over others was considered critical to our place in the world. Though we may not have realized it at the time, such a role limited our emotional lives, since any other expression might have created a break in the hegemonic view of masculinity and what its means to be a man, only highlighting and emphasizing our differences.

There is no doubt that almost all of us gay men were swathed in blue as babies and were given trucks and train sets on birthdays and holidays, when we might have preferred an EZ Bake Oven or My Little Pony. (I myself had hope that one day a Barbie would appear wrapped under the Christmas tree.) In effect, the messages we receive about being a boy are no different than those that any other boy receives, but we are, in fact, not like most other boys. As a result, young gay men find even greater conflict in their lives as they seek to reconcile these misunderstood, yet evolving, same-sex desires with imaging and massaging that clearly defines "being a man" in a way that is perhaps different from what they are feeling internally.

Confused about these desires and his identity, as a young teen Lorenzo thought he needed to "look" like a woman to be with a man:

> At that time I didn't hear nothing about one man being with another man. You heard about man being with a woman, so I thought that if I dressed up like a woman, I could have sexual relations with a man. I was 14, and it was just like one time I put on my mother's wig. I put on a pair of tight pants and and my mother's a big woman, so I would get her bras and fill them the best way I can. Well, if— maybe I had big titties, then they'll be more attracted to me. So, I used to sneak out late at night, sneak out the back door and just like walk up and down the streets, seeing if I could find some guy and, you know. I wasn't really sure what I was sup- posed to do at the time, until some guy showed me, and you know, so that's how I got started. You now, just whoring up and down the streets, you know.

In the photojournalistic essay "The Future of Masculinity Looks Like This,"[4] photographer Nate Jones decries these hegemonic conceptions of mascu- linity: "To most people in our world, masculinity has been characterized by heterosexuality, stoicism, athleticism, sexual activity, and overall domi- nance. But such a rigid definition of masculinity is toxic." For gay men this toxicity is quite palpable, especially when they're still learning about them- selves and their sexual identity. Tom vividly describes this reality:

> When I was 13 years old, I was bullied. We had a section that we traveled with through the whole day, so I couldn't get away from them. We were all in the same class. Um, and they would make fun of me. I wasn't quite sure why they were making fun of me, but it hurt. [They would say], "Oh, you know, "he's"—we didn't use the word "queer" or "faggot." Those weren't in vogue, uh, in the '60s, but, making fun of me in a way, made me feel feminine—effeminate. We had, in those years, things called slam books, and you'd pass those around, and there were all kinds of questions, and, you know, so you answered them, and I remember looking at it on my page, and several people had written "sissy." You know, and that really hurt.

In a similar vein, Wilson recalls his mother asking, "Are you a sissy?" to which he replied with a sense of pride, "I am a homosexual." Whether res- olute like Wilson or more vulnerable like Tom, being called a "sissy," or other homophobic slurs to demean one's manhood, is a painful reality. This type of pain haunts many of us throughout our lives as we reconcile what it means to be a man who also has sex with other men.

The perpetuation of this toxic masculinity, in which "manliness" is equated with physical and psychological domination, is built on a false notion that the concept of masculinity is so fragile that it would be undermined by any characteristic or behavior not aligned with man as the prototypical hunter-gatherer. These conceptions also permeate the gay male population. As the rights of women in the United States have progressed, there has been an accompanying change in female roles and a greater presence of women in traditionally male roles. Men, on the other hand, continue to resist professions that have long been considered "feminine," such as an elementary school teacher or a nurse, in fear of societal prejudices (think about Ben Stiller, who plays a nurse in the film *Meet the Parents*). In the meantime, though there have been advances in gay men's rights, there has not been an accompanying redefinition of masculinity.

Masculinity in the gay male community has also been conflated with sexual roles (receptive partners are less masculine), the pitch of one's voice (high voices are more feminine), and physique (muscularity is synonymous with masculinity). Such societal limitations create another level of burden for gay men as they struggle to come to grips with their sexuality and to be open about their sexuality to the world. In turn, some hide under hypermasculine shells to avoid coming out. Jeremy, a member of the Queer Generation, explains:

> Masculinity is definitely a big reason why a lot of gay men haven't found their identities. I still have a lot to learn about who I am as a gay man and I am now 26 years old.

Whether within or outside the gay community, gay men have historically had a unique relationship with masculinity, leading to the process of covering and passing as straight, adopted by some gay men, and toxic behavior including shaming of groups or individuals within the LGBTQ community. No matter what it may be called—the four terms "hegemonic masculinity," "hypermasculinity," "toxic masculinity, " and "masculinity so fragile" can be used interchangeably—the traditional power-based conception of masculinity and manliness has incessantly permeated society from time in memoriam. Even though there has been an evolution of this social construction over time, particularly within the Queer Generation, without being checked, this toxic form of masculinity rooted in power and privilege will perpetuate in all parts of American society, as was so clearly evidenced in the Supreme Court nomination hearings of Brett Kavanaugh.

CONCEPTUALIZING MASCULINITY

As noted by the Australian sociologist R. W. Connell, gay men are not excluded from embodying masculinity,[5] but they are often forced to negotiate their masculinity in various contexts: in their identities as gay men, in their desire of members of the same sex, and in how they present themselves to heterosexual men and women. Social structures create a struggle for gay men as they attempt to reconcile their identities and these contexts, including within the gay community itself, challenging their masculinity in both direct and indirect manners.[6]

Throughout the decades and across generations, gay men have had difficulties in owning their masculinity, as they have been considered weak and effeminate by a discriminatory and prejudicial society. Preconceived notions and the status quo have made it impossible for "sissy" men to be considered "real" men. This concept comes from years of misinformed findings by predominantly heterosexual researchers portraying gay men's behavior as deviant, characterized by physical and emotional weakness. This idea burrowed into the American consciousness for decades, setting gay men apart as emotionally ungrounded and feminine—the opposite of the "typical," heterosexual guy.

This level of intolerance has existed in most social settings, including in places of work, for decades, leading gay men to avoid coming out in certain contexts and to hide their true identity, as noted by Tom:

And I went to Columbia University, I did well there, and somehow talked myself into a job as an investment banker, and I joined the firm, now defunct, and went deeply back into the closet—well, at work, with people at work, because in all my years as an investment banker and I was at [the firm] 11 years before they blew up, and I didn't ever really meet someone that I knew for certain was gay. And it was a topic that was never discussed. When we did deals and you had to bring, a girlfriend with you, I took Mark's [his partner] sister. She was my beard. You know, I'd take her to these dinners, we were expected to show up with a woman. So, that—you know, it was—you know, I adopted a persona, and—as opposed to the authentic me—and I was—at some point, I got so confused. I didn't know which was which. You know, because I was spending so many hours being—projecting this persona. Who was the real Thomas?

Not only was Tom denying himself but also he was playing into the misogynistic attitudes of the time, with these women at dinner functioning solely as "arm candy."

In a different context but similar in terms of the vilification of gay men, and women, Seth described one of his high school experiences:

> I actually tried out for the cheerleading squad but, when I auditioned, I auditioned like a dancer, not like a cheerleader, and the guy cheerleaders, you know, they were not, outwardly, visibly gay. But of course they completely rejected me because, you know, I was auditioning more like a girl than I would be for a guy.

This mindset continues to this day in the hegemonic conceptions of masculinity espoused by many heterosexual men, who seek to establish power and dominance while subverting women and others, such as gay men.[7] In this regard, Wilson said,

> One of the things that I know from youth is that heterosexual men who feel this way, who see us in this monolithic way, the minute you walk in the room . . . when you come in, they go, "He's gay." And [then] they go, "[Not me,] I'm a man."

This sense of loathing of unmasculine men drove Matt Cain, editor-in-chief of *Attitude*, to commission a "masculinity survey,"[8] asking 5,000 gay men about their experiences. He found that 69% said they'd "been made to feel less of a man for being gay, bisexual or queer." Disappointingly, though not surprisingly, 92% said they "think effeminate gay men are still made fun of in the mainstream media." Lastly, 68% said they've "been on the receiving end of homophobic abuse that has specifically ridiculed their femininity." Cain concluded[9] with a recollection that so many of us can relate to:

> Like so many gay men, I can remember the limp wrists, mincing walks and camp impressions the straight boys did of me at school—although these can function as insults only if they're based on an understanding that being female is somehow inferior to being male.

Sociologist Mike Donaldson explains[10] how heterosexual men are pushed toward homophobia by society's demands to conform to a hypermasculine ideal. Their homophobic views and actions are then rewarded through social support from others or through a reaffirmation of, and decrease in anxiety about, their own "manliness." As Donaldson describes, "In other words, male heterosexual identity is sustained and affirmed by hatred for, and fear of, gay men."

This heterosexual hegemonic masculinity emboldens physical aggression as a means of maintaining control[11] and as way to define straight men's "maleness."[12] This understanding—depicted in the lives of prehistoric man, when the biological male was the hunter-gatherer—provides fodder for heterosexual men to subjugate, violate, and victimize women, as well as physically, emotionally, and socially victimize gay men. As gay men work to understand their own masculinity, however, they too are not precluded from hegemonic conceptions. Homophobia, including internalized homophobia, is a key element of masculinity and unfortunately, internalized homophobia is a psychosocial state with which many gay men grapple. Coming out is one way to combat and undo the powerful workings of internalized homophobia, but our inability to effectively confront this state keeps us closeted or, even if out, to adopt the personality of a "macho man," as characterized in the Village People's 1978 disco hit.

MASCULINITY IN THE GAY COMMUNITY

The narrow conception of masculinity espoused by much of heterosexual society also exists within the gay community, creating levels of power within gay couples and resulting in the shaming of sissy boys, girly men, and/or sexual bottoms (i.e., receptive partners). In fact, gay men have absorbed stereotypical manifestations of manliness and dominance for decades, perpetuating the struggle for power with, or dominance over, other men in the world-at-large but also within the gay population itself. This adoption of hypermasculinity forms the basis for many gay men who define their masculinity by their sexual prowess, physical appearance, and social behavior.[13]

Explaining this rigidity in masculinity, Wilson said, "All my life, I have never been attracted to other gay men. You know? I've always been attracted to quote-unquote straight-acting men." And as a young man in the 1950s trying to negotiate his masculinity and sexuality vis-à-vis his attractions, Wilson shaped his behaviors:

And so, I thought that I had to be feminine. I was really old before I learned that society—no matter how feminine I was, they didn't see me as a girl, you know? It took me a long time to get that through my head. So, I got very nelly [effeminate] and—and I started swishing, carrying my books up in my arm.

In the 1980s, hypermasculine conceptions were heightened in response to the AIDS epidemic. At that time, the virus' affect on individuals, and the community as a whole, led to the propagation of an image of gay men as frail, weak, and sickly.[6,13] In response, "the buff agenda" of physical masculinity was propagated among gay men. This trend in muscularity began as a means of bolstering body image and achieving masculine norms that had been stripped from them by the portrayal of the stereotypical AIDS victim.[14–16] Over time, however, this drive for masculinity began undermining the health of individuals and the gay population.

The use and abuse of anabolic steroids became common,[17] and mental health issues ensued,[18] creating a complex mutually reinforcing system of physical, emotional, and psychosocial health conditions. In a 2016 article published by *The Guardian*, gay men themselves indicated that hypermasculinity interfered with their mental health, substance use,[19] and willingness to seek out help for these issues.

These complex health patterns are rooted in the homophobic experiences gay men endure throughout their lives, especially at a young age. Homonegativity, or the deleterious attitudes of society toward homosexuality, has been associated with dissatisfaction with multiple aspects of gay men's own appearance, including overall body image, muscularity, and body fat.[20] These findings further underscore how gay men may try to compensate feelings of worth in a homophobic world, setting the stage for the adoption of hegemonic masculine ideals—ideals that have spread throughout the gay community itself. Many young gay men, for example, face bullying at the hands of their peers over their physical appearance and acumen.

Though potentially harmful, the adoption of hegemonic masculinity by gay men is certainly understood. Many gay men of my generation lived by the motto "no pecs, no sex," which served as drive for muscularity and masculinity, forcing other members of the community to follow suit or be left out. Masculinity, informed by domination and power, may also fuel eroticism.[21] For the AIDS Generation, masculinity was defined as a social construction informed by sex, appearance, and social behavior, much like the tenets of the paperback *The Butch Manual* by Clark Henley. First published in 1982,[22] Henley's book provides a humorous yet critical commentary on masculinity among gay men informed by the belief that this hypermasculine desire of "butchness"—a traditional stereotypical masculine appearance embodied by the Marlboro Man, GI Joe, superheroes, and other rugged, physically strong men—is influenced by social condition:

Relax. No one was born Butch. People were born babies and promptly burst into tears, which was most un-Butch. Yet when some people grew up they became inescapably Butch, while others are still silting on the sidelines waiting for a miracle. Is it in the genes? Natural selection? Divine intervention? No. These people have done their homework. They have read the writing on the bathroom walls. They have followed the advice of the graffiti gurus. They've given people what they think the people want. They've gone Butch.

The satire is powerful and at the same time troubling, as it depicts the norms revered in segments of the gay population. These norms shape coming out experiences and the lives of gay men throughout their course of development.

Gay men's feelings of internalized homophobia undermine their self-worth, create uncertainty and insecurity, and may result in obstacles to disclosing one's identity. Such conditions are worsened, and feelings of inadequacy are bolstered, by the gay community's reverence of physical perfection, muscularity, and aggressiveness. Coupled with internalized homophobia, an even greater deterrent to coming out and self-actualization develops. It takes great courage to counteract these homophobic feelings that permeate our consciousness and then to come out in a community where physical perfection is venerated. Sadly, the gay community may add to the burdens of many young men when they first come out knowing that they are not all necessarily specimens of such physical perfection.

I know this experience of a demanding gay community all too well. As a young 18-year-old coming of age as a gay man, after coming out, I decided to venture into my first gay bar, The Eagle, in New York City. The bar, defined as leather-Levi joint, certainly attracted patrons who adhered to tenets of *The Butch Manual.* Not knowing any better, I arrived at the Eagle dressed as usual: skin-tight designer jeans, large blow-dried hair (likely with a mullet), and a purple shirt—after all, it was 1981. To my surprise, and disappointment, no one paid attention to me. I looked around the bar, took mental notes on the everyone's clothing, style, and even attitude, and then I took action, as so many gay men do when we are learning who we are. The next weekend I arrived at the bar sporting a buzzed hair cut, razor stubble, worn-down Levi's jeans, and combat boots—I was the belle of the ball. It took me decades to realize that I didn't need to be that person; I didn't need to only date men with facial hair or wear only Levi's 501s.

Though my first exposure to butch culture was almost 40 years ago, gay men struggled with the rigid conception of masculinity in the gay community even earlier as well. Capturing this idea with a touch of humor, Ryan, of the Stonewall Generation, said:

> *You know, we were no better than the straight people because probably the most prejudiced people in the world are straight white men. Excuse me. Probably the most prejudiced people in the world are gay white men.*

Today, these masculine expectations continue to be imposed on us in different environments and social contexts and are associated with aggression and the suppression of emotion, perpetuating the trauma we as gay men experience throughout our youth and adulthood. While sexual prejudice against gay men, as well as antifemininity, serve as sources of anger toward gay men by straight men,[23] this pattern is mimicked in the gay community itself. The oppressed becomes the oppressor.

Based on the survey in *Attitudes* mentioned earlier in the chapter, the *Gay Star News*[8] reported that among 5,000 survey respondents, 71% admitted they were actively turned off by a partner with typically feminine attributes, while 41% of respondents believed that "effeminate gay men give the gay community a bad image or reputation." Another question resulted in 41% responding that, "at some point they've thought they are less of a man because of their sexuality." The results of this survey show a vicious cycle in which gay men are treated negatively because of their supposed lack of masculinity, then internalize this negativity and apply it within the gay community, causing gay men to feel worse about themselves, their sexuality, and their manhood.

Sexual Role

One common point of contention in regard to masculinity within the gay community is an age-old question: Butch or dandy? Of course, the question in itself is ridiculous. Certainly most gay men do not squarely fit into this dichotomy, yet it is how we are portrayed outside and within our own community. Those gay men who adhere to this rigidity also clearly contend with "masculinity so fragile." The idea is perpetuated by the false dichotomization of "tops" and "bottoms"—in reference to sexual position—where bottoms are made to feel less worthy, much like women, because of their sexual roles. The issue has become so heated that, when writer Lamar Dawson released a list of 10 things that gay men should stop doing as part of their New Years' resolutions for 2018, the #1 item was "bottom-shaming."[24] Just as many of our identities exist on a spectrum including gender, research has supported the idea that our sexual roles are also fluid, particularly among younger gay men of the Queer Generation.[25]

In contrast, there is greater rigidity in the conceptions of masculinity and gender fluidity among the men of the AIDS and Stonewall generations due to the environment in which their gay identities developed—a time in which women, including lesbians, and in turn "effeminate" gay men were demeaned even more than they are today. This rigidity in gender roles was also apparent in Wilson's narrative:

> At that time, in Baltimore, there was this division in the subculture. You know, if two queens did not rub each other. That's what it was called. Like the lesbians. We used to say that they were "flattin'," "pancakin'," you know, because there was nothing—you can't—you know, they're flat. So, that's—we'd [say] things, "Oh girl, I don't flat," you know? So, that meant nothing could happen between us, you know, because both of us were nelly.

Gay men who insist that that they fit squarely and only into the category of top and nothing else fuel their own internalized homophobia, emboldening hegemonic masculinity that demonizes gay men who are considered bottoms. In doing so, these men are, in many ways, keeping part of themselves closeted. Even in Latino culture, in which the roles of *activo* and *pasivo* are steeped in the hypermasculine conception of *machismo*, emotions and circumstances play a critical role in shaping sexual roles and behaviors.[26] This is to say that even in a hypermasculine culture, a hypermasculine man may not always be sexually dominant, whereas in the United States there is too often, and especially among older men, a preoccupation in the gay community with masculinity and sexual role.

Unfortunately, for those who have lived these experiences, none of this information may come as a surprise, as it has been long documented. In the early 2000s, I conducted a series of studies examining and seeking to understand masculinity among gay men, particularly HIV-positive gay men, and developed a scale to assess conceptions of hegemonic masculinity.[13] The scales consists of three domains: "Masculinity as Sexual Behavior," "Masculinity as Appearance," and "Masculinity as Social Behavior," which were also found to be related to sexual adventurism and body image, risk taking, and substance use. The latter subscale of Social Behavior included these items, which were highly endorsed by samples of gay men:

- Drag queens undermine the idea of masculinity in the gay community.
- I am not comfortable around unmasculine gay men.
- I would not have sex with a masculine looking man who acted in any way feminine.
- A masculine man is "butch" in both behavior and appearance.

- I watch my behavior to make sure that I act masculine around other gay men.

These findings point to the dominance of stereotypical masculinity in the gay community and the value gay men place on their worth as defined by how the look and act, and with whom they socialize and have sex. Unfortunately, this mentality creates many missed opportunities for gay men who refuse to look beyond the hypermasculine ideal, whether that be a potential partner, a stronger community, or better understanding of one's self.

Race and sexual role are also often intersecting and are perpetuated by intrapersonal beliefs and cultural stereotypes. Myths exist within the gay community about all black men being masculine, dominant tops and Asian men being passive, feminine bottoms.[27] Such oversimplifications are replete with homophobia, racism, and hypermasculine conceptions. Ultimately for all gay men, regardless of class, race, ethnicity, and/or culture, sexual roles may be shaped by gender roles to the extent that a man espouses hypermasculinity. It has been found, however, that expectations of masculinity may even be heightened within gay male communities of color.

In a study of methamphetamine use among black gay men, the hegemonic views of black masculinity coupled with the objectification of black men by white men served as catalysts in the use of this drug in the gay community (the need for belonging both within the gay and black communities also played a role).[28] Fast-forward to a 2017 editorial by David-Butler Sims, the national president of the first intercollegiate fraternity for gay, bisexual, and progressive men, Delta Phi Upsilon, who emotionally pleaded with the black gay community to release its rigid conceptions of masculinity, which inflict great harm on black gay men's health:[29] "When we in the gay and black communities separate ourselves into groups of masculine and feminine and decry anyone who doesn't fit the heteronormative definition of a 'man' we create barriers for addressing the real problems we face and we buoy the hazardous and hurtful stereotypes the very segments we've created are trying to combat."

The circumstances surrounding hegemonic masculinity within the gay community may, however, be changing. Just as younger gay men are embracing fluidity in sexual and gender identities, they are also doing so with sexual roles.[30] The hope of undoing this toxic masculinity rests with a new generation, the Queer Generation, who have collectively begun to engage in an open and honest dialogue around the meanings of masculinity, questioning "traditions" and norms both within and outside the gay community.[31] As this new generation forges a more inclusive community, embracing less rigid and more fluid perspectives, it's also developing more ideal circumstance for coming out. When roles and expectation are less rigidly defined, both within the gay community and society at large, it is less challenging for individuals to be who they are, and in effect it is more possible and permissible to come out into the world with all aspects of identity intact.

THE EVOLUTION OF MASCULINITY

Just as the Queer Generation is taking a new approach to many aspects of what it means to be a gay man today, it is also taking a new approach toward masculinity. Many members seem to understand and experience gender and masculinity in a more expansive manner. The men of the Queer Generation are clear and vocal in their repudiation of hegemonic masculinity and how conceptions of the fragility of masculinity are undermining the gay community. Miguel astutely summarized these ideas:

> I think in a dialogue that's currently happening now—people are examining masculinity—not just straight men but gay men as well. Like how it promotes, you know, like, how most versions of masculinity are toxic, and how, like, they promote misogyny and trans misogyny and, like, racism, like, all kinds of terrible things that need to be addressed within the whole concept of masculinity.

Miguel also discussed the dangers and privilege associated with his own masculinity:

> I am hyper aware of [the toxicity of hypermasculinity]. So I have to, you know, tone it back a little bit, and like, or I have to make sure that I'm not oppressing anyone. I'm not trying to [be masculine when I'm assertive] because a lot of versions of masculinity involve, being aggressive, domineering. And sometimes you need to learn how to scale back [your assertiveness], and especially to, for the benefit of not just yourself but also for others.

Yasar also noted the prevalence and dangers of hypermasculinity, especially within the black population, the same issues David-Butler Sims pointed out. Recall that Yasar is a large muscular man who also sports beautiful bright yellow painted nails:

> I feel like when I'm around like black men, we can get into like masculinity issues, and like toxic masculinity. Just not knowing what's going to happen. As you can see, I'm a bigger guy, like buffer guy. So a lot of times I don't get like that side eye or

that slack. Or I get side eyes but I don't get like people harassing me or anything.
Because like sometimes they'll see the way I'm built and they'll see my nails or
they'll see something that presents—they see as feminine and they'll be like, "Oh
what's going on there?" I don't know what goes through their minds.

As a result, depending on the situation, Yasar hides aspects of who he is: "I tend to cover up my nails or like have a deeper voice or not say certain things." Jeremy also notes how he changes his own behavior as a result of societal pressures:

There are still times where I find myself holding back my true self because there are
straight men around and I don't want to come off too gay. I feel a lot of us gay men
deal with those type of issues due to how society views the LGBTQ community.

Jeremy's hesitance is also rooted in the messages he received growing up in a Latino culture:

When I was 11, I knew I was having thoughts about boys and that I found some
of my boy friends attractive at school, but within my Dominican culture being gay
was wrong. Throughout my childhood, and as I became older, a lot of my own
family members talked bad about those few men that were out in our Spanish
communities and in Dominican Republic itself. They would call them different de-
rogatory names and so I grew up thinking being gay was wrong.

So, too, Reid demonstrated a keen awareness of the dangers of hypermasculinity as they relate to gay men, which he developed at a young age, though not just within the gay community. He relayed this story about his adolescence, before he came out to his father:

I used to watch, like, Queer Eye for the Straight Guy or Queer as Folk and my
dad, my dad is a stereotypical Midwestern, like, 6'5", 350, big guy. "I love my guns,
I love hunting, I love masculinity, I love working out." I would watch these shows,
and he would walk past the living room and be like, "If I ever see these faggots, I'm
gonna fucking shoot them."

Older gay men of the AIDS Generation also share some awareness and concern over hypermasculinity, albeit much more limited than members of the Queer Generation, whose consciousness is razor-sharp focused on this issue. Emilio, of the AIDS Generation, noted,

> I think my thoughts of what it means to be a gay man have changed as I've become more self-aware. So back then [when I first came out], I was only into masculine guys. Gay men had to be masculine. I didn't like flamey queens, where now, I have friends who are fem, drag queens, trans, gay, butch, queen, whatever, the lipstick lesbian, you know. I have so much—so much of a variety in my life of what G—LGBTQ is that my mind is open, so I'm more open about what it means. Whereas back then, when I had the shame and the guilt and, you know, the self-loathing, I had a different version.

A lack of acceptance of other gay men who may have been deemed "feminine," or not masculine enough, by Emilio in his early life perpetuated intolerance within the community and potentially interfered with Emilio's opportunity to meet substantial and wonderful men. This rigid sense of manliness is a further manifestation of self-loathing fueled by internalized homophobia. Hypermasculinity is in some ways a means of "being a man" while being out and may function to alleviate the burdens of being gay—ultimately another way of fitting in.

In the interviews conducted, of all the men from the AIDS Generation, it is Seth who most vehemently aligned his perspectives with those of the younger men in regard to hypermasculine attitudes:

> I sort of get lumped into being gay because I feel, as I've grown and come to experience other men who I feel are similar to me, not just gay, but men who love men who also identify as pseudo-psychic, fairy, what have you, um, queer, that there's some part of our nature that—or at least the subset that I identify with—that–have a fuller sense of being than, I think, a lot of hetero people. I think we live at sort of the crux of where spirit and matter exist, and um, I like walking that way. I feel like it's a privilege, and it's also a responsibility.

Seth's alignment of the fairy, queer ethos is a counter to the tenets of the hypermasculine norm, as he assigns himself emotions that are more traditionally feminine. However, it is interesting to note his appearance is still that of a butch male: muscular, bearded, and with cropped hair.

The awareness of the dangers of hypermasculinity, and the articulation of the tenets associated with it, is seen much less among the Stonewall Generation. In fact, during the interviews for this book, the concept was all but absent from its members' narratives. This pattern is not surprising, as such nuanced and intricate understandings have only been made possible by the advances gay men have made in securing their rights. The men of the Stonewall Generation came of age in a landscape in which being gay was both a crime and a pathology, viewed as an abomination and a disease.

Little emotional and cognitive space existed at the time for disentangling the meanings of masculinity and manliness. For the men of the AIDS Generation, the awareness is relatively recent, having managed to survive an era in which most all of our thoughts were directed toward defeating a virus.

It is the Queer Generation that leads our newest battle in deconstructing the monolithic conception of what it means to be gay and to be a man. These efforts are also paving the way for the evolution of a more all encompassing and accepting community, where gender and sexuality are fluidly defined, where being a man and being masculine may manifest in many different ways, and where coming out will become less burdensome for the high-pitched, skinny man, who likes to be, and takes pride in being, a bottom.

Covering and Passing

Though there is no doubt an evolution taking place in how gay men think about masculinity, even nowadays many gay men rely on their masculinity to cover their gay identity. Passing and covering are processes undertaken to hide one's identity, or identities, by marginalized groups as means of advancement, survival, and management of the stigma that they experience, as noted by sociologist Erving Goffman in his seminal work, *Stigma: Notes on the Management of Spoiled Identity*.[32] For gay men, covering their sexuality, or attempting to "pass as straight," often relies on hegemonic masculinity. For those who are also members of nonwhite racial and ethnic groups, covering may also extend to their racial or ethnic identities. No matter what identity it is applied to, covering is a denial of one's self that perpetuates feelings of otherness.

In the recent past, portrayals of gay life and gay men as ill, villainous, or deranged have been an impetus for covering. These depictions come from a misunderstanding, or lack of empathy, abut the gay experience, such as the ravages of AIDS. While accurately shown in films like *Longtime Companion* and *An Early Frost*, such onscreen portraits of the disease would be enough to keep any young gay man in the closet, in fear of potential physical and emotional destruction caused by making love with another man. Other movies that attempt to describe and share the difficulties of being a gay man fail to do so accurately, relying on ascribed Hollywood stereotypes, as noted in the 1995 documentary *The Celluloid Closet* (based on the book of the same name by Vito Russo), which deciphers how the mainstream entertainment industry has played such an outsized role in the perceptions of LGBTQ people. And even in the play *Boys in the Band*, written by a gay man, life is depicted as toxic and difficult. In reviewing the 2018 production, *New York Times* critic Ben Brantley writes:[33]

I was a 13-year-old North Carolina middle-school student then, and secretly followed the coverage of what became a Cultural Event with an uneasy fascination. Though I hadn't read the play, all accounts of it suggested that no one in his right mind would want to grow up to be like the miserable and vicious misfits it depicted. In his original New York Times review, Clive Barnes spoke of "the special self-dramatization and the frightening self-pity—true I suppose of all minorities, but especially true of homosexuals." And I thought that was just how teenagers were! I got myself a (temporary) girlfriend, pronto.

Such social, including familial, conditions during adolescence provided ample fuel to cover for Brantley and many of the older gay men we interviewed. In fact, Tom, a contemporary of Brantley's, covered well into his adult life. After his father passed away, Tom found himself employing this technique once again while with his mother when they were trying access his father's military benefits:

[During the interview at the VA, the administrator] asked me where I lived, and I guess I had put down as the contact person my boyfriend; so when he asked me, "What's his address?" I gave him the same address, of course, because we live together, and there was this silence for a moment. And he said, "Oh, you just live in different apartments," and I didn't—I didn't contradict him. I didn't correct him. And, my mother was sitting, like, over there, and she gave me this look, and I couldn't tell whether it was, "Go on, tell him," or—I think it was, "Let's just let sleeping dogs lie," and it gets me even now that I was a coward—I was too afraid to tell this guy that I'm gay, and, yeah, he's living at the same address, and he also sleeps in the same bed with me, and we also have sex together.

Despite advances in conceptions of masculinity, passing and covering have been used even among the youngest of men interviewed for this book. Although he possesses a high level of self-awareness regarding hypermasculinity, Miguel nonetheless also recognizes the advantages of hegemonic masculinity as a way to get by in a homophobic world:

I can pass for straight if I need to. I don't find a problem in it. I think that passing for myself is a privilege that I use to my own advantage because I feel like if you have it, why not? Use it. Use it in a more moral sense. I feel like if I have this privilege to pass, then I can provide a level of protection for people who don't.

Miguel's use of hypermasculinity as means of survival seems to provide him and other gay men physical, if not psychological, protection. Still he is steadfast and clear in his understanding of the processes he is enacting and why:

> My ability to pass allows also for me to infiltrate places that wouldn't allow other people who were not cis males who were passing. So for instance, like, a lot of opportunities for DJs and musicians and stuff only get passed along from certain men to men, the boys club. Um, and it's usually, like, you know, I scratch your back, you scratch mine kind of thing. We put each other on and we build a, a prefabricated notion of success. I can infiltrate that because I'm a man, so I—and whatever I do will be 100 times more valued than if I was, you know, a woman or a queer person.

He uses the doors that are opened for him—doors that may have remained closed if he were to have come out to those same people who allowed him access—to help others who are barred from a social setting, job, or opportunity because of their race or gender identity:

> But within these opportunities that have been presented to me, I can still pass those opportunities on to people of color, to people of, to queer people, to trans people who don't have those opportunities. I can open up doors and keep those doors open. So and to better, better diversify my industry right now, so it's like a lot of musicians, men, women, and trans people, and, like, uh, people from all sort of diverse backgrounds. Like, they won't get these opportunities, but I can at least try to get them for them. And I can kind of step back on my own and kind of just be like, okay, so I don't really need this, but you totally do. You should take this.

In his 2006 book *Covering: The Assault on Our Civil Rights*,[34] legal scholar and gay man Kenji Yoshino examined the extent to which racial and ethnic minorities modulate their identities in order to be accepted and integrated into mainstream American culture. This idea is rooted in the assimilation that many immigrants felt forced to undertake in order to make their way in the United States. Gay men also cover in order to advance. In fact Yoshino wrote about this situation in academia, stating:[35]

> When I began teaching at Yale Law School in 1998, a friend spoke to me frankly. "You'll have a better chance at tenure," he said, "if you're a homosexual professional than if you're a professional homosexual." Out of the closet for six years at the time, I knew what he meant. To be a "homosexual professional" was to be a professor of constitutional law who "happened" to be gay. To be a "professional homosexual" was to be a gay professor who made gay rights his work. Others echoed

the sentiment in less elegant formulations. Be gay, my world seemed to say. Be openly gay, if you want. But don't flaunt.

I fully understand where Yoshino is coming from, as I, too, had to make a conscious decision when I entered academia to lead with being gay. As I noted in an interview in 2017,[36] being a LGBTQ person in higher education and exhibiting only a small amount of your identity is much different than making LGBTQ identity the cornerstone of your work, such as I have with LGBTQ health.

Yet even in my full actualized life, I still occasionally find myself covering. I recall a car ride back from my apartment to midtown Manhattan, when my Uber driver, a young immigrant man, spoke to me about his wife and children, and the importance of having children. He asked if I was married and if I had children of my own. I told him, yes, I was married but with no children. He then insisted that my wife and I must have children—I didn't clarify or correct him. That day, I was wearing a baseball cap, jeans, and a wrinkled, unkempt t-shirt, and I had a scruffy unshaven beard and the must of an "un-showered" guy—the hallmark of a "man's man"—so I was passing. But I was also covering. Even at 55, despite who I am, the work I've done, and my openness about my sexuality, my internalized homophobia is still very much a part of me, albeit a smaller one than decades ago, and something that I know is engrained and maybe inescapable.

Though in most instances covering is less common today in the United States due to societal advances, it still takes place, even among the men of the Queer Generation. Jeremy's need to hide his sexual identity from his family, for example, was only reinforced during his youth:

I began covering being gay at the age of 11 years old. Family members would push me to like girls and asked me questions such as if I had a girlfriend in school or if I liked any girls. This heavy pressure I received from my family forced me to believe that my thoughts about boys were wrong and that I had to cover being gay as much as possible. Through the years of 11 to 17 there were times I hated myself for fantasizing about boys. I would cry at night because all I wanted to be was "normal," and I definitely didn't want to disappoint my family. During those same years I forced myself to have girlfriends as well as have sex with girls. At the time I was very confused of whether I was actually enjoying being with girls and whether I was ever going to forget these thoughts about being with boys.

Just like the feelings Jeremy had as he got older, covering becomes even less tolerable for older men as they emerge into their adulthood and middle age. Nonetheless, covering and passing continues to be a method employed by gay men to cope with the world around them, projecting a stereotype of masculinity that may not be true to who they are. This form of denial may come from a desire to keep the peace within one's family, but it is ultimately about the inability to negotiate sexuality with male identity, leading to a lack of self-acceptance.

Even in environments where openness and inclusion might be expected, it's still not a given that gay men will feel comfortable disclosing their sexual identity. For example, despite his immersion in the theater, Emilio covered at different times in various contexts:

> I covered being gay throughout college and into my opening of Miss Saigon on Broadway. I dated a woman in college whom I proposed to. Thank God she said no. Post college, my mother and father, my sister and brother-in-law came to town for my opening on Broadway. During the early evening while I hung out with them, gold medal figure skater, Katarina Witt was my date. Once my parents and everyone else left, I spent the rest of the evening with my second date, Jerry Mitchell. It made me feel guilt and shame. I mainly did it because I thought that what was expected of me by my strict Catholic mother.

As he shared this story, it also became clear that covering was also related to Emilio's challenging negotiation of his own masculinity and hypermasculine conceptions:

> When I first came out I was very judgmental about effeminate gay men. As I went through therapy I realized it was my own internal homophobia and my failure to accept my feminine side. I wanted to play the macho Latino.

Sadly, even after a lifetime of gay identity development, many of us rely on these behaviors in difficult situations, or in moments of fear and isolation, almost as a reflex. As Tom says, "I think, to my dying day, I think there will still be parts of me, where I don't—where I'm a coward, where I will cover again."

FINAL THOUGHTS

The language and attitudes of hypermasculinity are so engrained in our society, that they many times go unnoticed or are simply accepted as the norm. While watching the US figure skating championships, a prelude to the selection of the team for the 2018 Winter Olympic Games in PyeongChang, South Korea, I was excited to see Adam Rippon compete. Rippon, the

2016 US men's figure skating champion, is the first openly gay American Olympic figure skater, which he revealed in an interview by stating, "The first time I kissed a boy, I'm like, 'I definitely am gay' "[37]—a feeling so many of us can understand.

Throughout the competition, the commentators described Rippon as "sassy," "wearing his heart on his sleeve," and "effervescent." Rather than acknowledging Rippon's sexual identity, they chose instead to use coded terms that, though they may have functioned as codes for gay, were actually microaggressions targeting gay men and the LGBTQ population at large. Such expressions may not be surprising when made my heterosexual cisgender man like Terry Gannon, one of the commentators, but Johnny Weir, a figure skating champion and gay man himself, made such statements as well. Though neither likely meant to support the vitriol of hegemonic masculinity, they certainly illuminated it. Fortunately, Adam Rippon's words and actions during and after the Olympics normalized his gay identity in a beautiful and calm way—he didn't need to scream, "I'm gay"; he just was and is.

This anecdote demonstrates the crux of the dilemma with regard to hegemonic masculinity. At times, hypermasculinity seems to be inescapable whether outside or within the gay community. Fortunately such statements and actions are countered in recent times by more enlightened views. In the documentary *Freedom*, British comedian Rickey Gervais demonstrated a clear understanding of the struggles of gay men with regard to masculinity when he jokingly described George Michael as a gay man who states very clearly and loudly "I have a cock"—an opposition to societal views of gay men as dandies and fairies if there ever was one. Still, society is accepting so long as we don't flaunt our sexual prowess, as was the case with Liberace, the gay couple in the film *The Birdcage*, or as is currently the case with the guys on *Queer Eye*. Such stereotypical depictions of gay men are safe for America—as long as we are eunuchs all is good. But when two dudes kiss and hold hands and take pride in their maleness, that sends many Americans into a tailspin.

Ultimately, despite the advances in society and LGBTQ rights, homophobia is very much part of our culture and our lives. And it is this homophobia that directs and shapes ongoing hegemonic masculinity targeting gay men and then being weaponized by gay men within their community, perpetuating the ills of society at large. It is no wonder that many gay men therefore sidestep speaking their truth publicly, avoiding sexual disclosure in circumstances where they feel that it's either safer or more advantageous to cover or pass. In doing so, they deny themselves and their identity, a situation that is even more complex for gay men of color, who also need to reconcile their gay identity and their racial and/or ethnic identities in an attempt to integrate all aspects of who they are, both with communities of color and society at large.

REFERENCES

1. Newman BS, Muzzonigro PG. The effects of traditional family values on the coming out process of gay male adolescents. *Adolescence.* 1993;28(109):213–226.
2. Hammond WP. Taking it like a man: masculine role norms as moderators of the racial discrimination–depressive symptoms association among African American men. *Am J Public Health.* 2012;102 Suppl 2:S232–S241.
3. Oliffe JL, Kelly MT, Bottorff JL, Johnson JL, Wong ST. "He's more typically female because he's not afraid to cry": connecting heterosexual gender relations and men's depression. *Soc Sci Med.* 2011;73(5):775–782.
4. Jones N. The future of masculinity looks like this. *Very Good Light* 2017.
5. Connell RW. A very straight gay: masculinity, homosexual experience, and the dynamics of gender. *Am Sociol Rev.* 1992;57(6):735–751.
6. Halkitis PN. An exploration of perceptions of masculinity among gay men living with HIV. *J Mens Stud.* 2001;9(3):413–429.
7. Connell RW, Messerschmidt JW. Hegemonic masculinity: rethinking the concept. *Gend Soc.* 2005;19(6):829–859.
8. Besanvalle J. Almost three quarters of the gay community have been turned off by feminine men, new survey finds. *Gay Star News* 2017.
9. Cain M. What gay men's attitudes to masculinity have taught me about womanhood. *The Guardian* 2017.
10. Donaldson M. What is hegemonic masculinity? *Theory Soc.* 1993;22(5):643–657.
11. Sijtsema JJ, Veenstra R, Lindenberg S, Salmivalli C. Empirical test of bullies' status goals: assessing direct goals, aggression, and prestige. *Aggress Behav.* 2009;35(1):57–67.
12. Krug EG, Mercy JA, Dahlberg LL, Zwi AB. The world report on violence and health. *Lancet.* 2002;360(9339):1083–1088.
13. Halkitis PN, Green KA, Wilton L. Masculinity, body image, and sexual behavior in HIV-seropositive gay men: a two-phase formative behavioral investigation using the Internet. *Int J Mens Health.* 2004;3(1):27–42.
14. Brewster ME, Sandil R, DeBlaere C, Breslow A, Eklund A. "Do you even lift, bro?" Objectification, minority stress, and body image concerns for sexual minority men. *Psychol Men Masc.* 2017;18(2):87.
15. DeBlaere C, Brewster ME. A confirmation of the Drive for Muscularity Scale with sexual minority men. *Psychol Sex Orientat Gend Divers.* 2017;4(2):227.
16. Yelland C, Tiggemann M. Muscularity and the gay ideal: body dissatisfaction and disordered eating in homosexual men. *Eat Behav.* 2003;4(2):107–116.
17. Halkitis PN, Moeller RW, DeRaleau LB. Steroid use in gay, bisexual, and nonidentified men-who-have-sex-with-men: relations to masculinity, physical, and mental health. *Psychol Men Masc.* 2008;9(2):106.
18. Fischgrund BN, Halkitis PN, Carroll RA. Conceptions of hypermasculinity and mental health states in gay and bisexual men. *Psychol Men Masc.* 2012;13(2):123.
19. Marsh S, Guardian readers. "As boys, we are told to be brave": men on masculinity and mental health. *The Guardian* 2016.
20. Siconolfi DE, Kapadia F, Moeller RW, et al. Body dissatisfaction in a diverse sample of young men who have sex with men: the P18 Cohort Study. *Arch Sex Behav.* 2016;45(5):1227–1239.

21. Velasquez-Manoff M. Real men get rejected, too. *New York Times* 2018.

22. Henley C. *The butch manual: The current drag and how to do it.* New York: New American Library; 1982.

23. Parrott DJ, Peterson JL, Vincent W, Bakeman R. Correlates of anger in response to gay men: effects of male gender role beliefs, sexual prejudice, and masculine gender role stress. *Psychol Men Masc.* 2008;9(3):167.

24. Dawson L. 10 things gay men should stop doing in 2018. *Logo New Now Next* 2017.

25. Johns MM, Pingel E, Eisenberg A, Santana ML, Bauermeister J. Butch tops and femme bottoms? Sexual positioning, sexual decision making, and gender roles among young gay men. *Am J Mens Health.* 2012;6(6):505–518.

26. Carballo-Diéguez A, Dolezal C, Nieves L, Díaz F, Decena C, Balan I. Looking for a tall, dark, macho man . . . : sexual-role behaviour variations in Latino gay and bisexual men. *Cult Health Sex.* 2004;6(2):159–171.

27. Lick DJ, Johnson KL. Intersecting race and gender cues are associated with perceptions of gay men's preferred sexual roles. *Arch Sex Behav.* 2015;44(5):1471–1481.

28. Jerome RC, Halkitis PN. Stigmatization, stress, and the search for belonging in black men who have sex with men who use methamphetamine. *J Black Psychol.* 2009;35(3):343–365.

29. Butler-Sims D. The gay community's obsession with "masculinity" is killing us. *Huffington Post* 2017

30. Pachankis JE, Buttenwieser IG, Bernstein LB, Bayles DO. A longitudinal, mixed methods study of sexual position identity, behavior, and fantasies among young sexual minority men. *Arch Sex Behav.* 2013;42(7):1241–1253.

31. Schuessler L. What is masculinity? One trans man's journey to self-discovery. *The Good Men Project* 2018.

32. Goffman E. Stigma: notes on a spoiled identity. New York: Simon & Schuster; 1963.

33. Brantley B. Review: Jim Parsons and Zachary Quinto enter sniping in "The Boys in the Band." *New York Times* 2018.

34. Yoshino K. *Covering: The hidden assault on our civil rights.* New York: Random House Trade Paperbacks; 2007.

35. Yoshino K. The pressure to cover. *New York Times* 2006.

36. Verbanas P. Openly gay university dean seeks to shatter perceptions, improve LGBTQ health. *Rutgers Today* 2017.

37. Buzinski J. American skater will be among group of first openly gay male Winter Olympians at Pyeongchang 2018. *Out Sports* 2018.

CHAPTER 7

Intersectionality and Racism

The website www.homohistory.com is an online archive containing a multitude of photos of gay men and lesbians from throughout history. The images on the site are powerful, beautiful, and haunting, pictures from the past expressing the sepia-toned love stories between men and between women across time and generations. Though many such photos have likely been destroyed or hidden away, those that have been uncovered and shared act as another strong piece of the lesbian, gay, bisexual, transgender, and queer (LGBTQ) history, reminders of those who have come before us, some who were proud of their sexual identities and some who felt they needed to cover their true selves from the rest of the world. Behind each photo is an unknown life history, many of which will remain unknown, but continue to inspire, challenge, and create a sense of wonder.

Unfortunately, these photos are also demonstrative of the painful reality of the gay community, and that of American society writ large: namely, the segregation and racism embedded in US history and culture. It is nearly impossible to find an image on the site that depicts gay men of different races, cultures, or ethnicities together in one photograph. The images show individuals and couples who are practically doppelgangers of each other, much like the nearly all white cast of *Friends* or *Girls*, whose main characters, despite living in New York City in the 1990s and 2010s respectively, socialize almost exclusively with individuals of the same skin tone. The images bring to light major challenges that we face as a society as we define who we are, namely intersectionality and racism, both of which shape the coming out process for gay men.

The ideas of intersectionality and racism may seem diametrically opposed, as intersectionality honors our differences, while racism, of course, does not. Our perspectives dictate much of how we view and experience these social conditions, just like whether a glass is half full or half empty. In many instances the multiple identities gay men hold—as lover, brother, father, man, sexual minority, and the rest—are a celebration of intersectionality, ones that are honored and considered dear. However, in an increasingly hostile and polarized society—a large portion of which seeks to "otherize" all but cisgender heterosexual white males—owning multiple identities, especially in regard to race, sexuality, and gender, creates an opportunity for the venom of hate to emerge, as sadly witnessed in Charlottesville, Virginia, in the summer of 2017. That August, a group of right-wing, conservative white straight men, including white supremacists and neo-Nazis, took to the streets for a "Unite the Right" protest, where they railed against immigrants, people of color, religious minorities, and the LGBTQ community, resulting in the death of one counterprotester who was run over by a car.

Yasar's words perfectly encapsulate the current sociopolitical conditions that sexual, gender, and racial minorities face as they simply try to live fully integrated lives:

As far as like my identity goes my queer identity, it's not as bad. It's not really as bad, but then like when you're including that with my blackness it's been pretty rough considering a lot of trans women, black trans women [are] being killed, being slaughtered, honestly. Like I think the 23rd trans woman was killed recently. Like two weeks ago.

Intersectionality informs the ongoing and evolving understanding that "a gay man is not a gay man is not a gay man." Rather each gay man holds multiple identities that reflect his own understanding of his race, ethnicity, culture, class, and myriad other aspects of being, including his gender identity and sexual identity.[1] A core component of intersectional theory is that these identities do not exist in isolation but rather work together to shape how an individual thinks of himself and experiences life. In other words, race does not exist separately from sexual identity or class or gender identity; rather these identities interact and shape the realties and life conditions of a person—and these identities cannot easily be split apart. In this regard, New York City–based author Morgan Jerkins states,[2] "I can't slice away at my identity as though it was made up of individuals parts." No one can: though they are rarely considered in relation to each other, the identities we hold are woven together with intricate stitches.

To understand the totality of lives and intersectional identities in the LGBTQ community, it's imperative to consider how these identities interact and shape the privileges and challenges members face, both within and outside the community. There is evidence that suggests people's multiple identities, when viewed as subordinate to the "dominant" group, bestow a disadvantage,[1] leading to intersectional invisibility, not being seen or heard, within society.[3] In turn, this invisibility impacts a great many aspects of gay men's lives, including their ability to successfully come our and their health.

In a powerful op-ed,[4] Daryl Hannah, a black gay man, explained how his own race and sexual identity have shaped his decision to not take the anti-viral Truvada as PrEP, an HIV prevention strategy. This decision is, in part, a result of his mistrust of the medical community, stemming from a lack of health professional's understanding of the specific issues that affect both the African American community and the gay community. These health-care providers often fail to acknowledge that their patients are complex mosaics shaped by social circumstances; that they are not simply biological organisms affected solely by pathogens. A biopsychosocial perceptive is therefore integral to define health and wellness—a paradigm recognizing that biological phenomena interact with behavioral and emotional states and social conditions to shape a person's overall well-being. Simply put: health must also be understood in an intersectional way.

Similarly, Miguel summarized the underpinnings of intersectionality and the associated struggles:

> The black lived gay experience is a way different experience than the Latino gay experience versus the white gay experience versus the Asian gay experience. They're all totally different.

This difference in experience may be nowhere more apparent than in the act of disclosing sexual identity, as multiple intersectional identities inform and direct the coming out process.

RACE, ETHNICITY, CULTURE, AND CLASS

Psychologist Margaret Rosario has conducted extensive work on LGBTQ identity in communities of color. Through her research, Rosario found that while developmental milestones associated with emerging into adolescence and young adulthood were similar across races and ethnicities, numerous other differences exist.[5] Notably, both black and Latino sexual minority youth disclose their sexual identities to fewer people than their white peers. This hesitance to come out indicates that young gay men of color may be less likely to receive the full range of social support than white gay men when disclosing their sexual identity. These circumstances may in part exist because young ethnic minority gay men struggle to negotiate affiliation and loyalty to both their ethnic community and the gay community.[6] This patterns is also true for many first-generation gay men, whose immigrant families often adhere to "traditional" cultural tenets. For many, this pull between the two results in the rejection of one community over the other for a period of time, normally the ethnic community as means of forming their gay identity. Later in life, many of these same men seek to reconcile and negotiate both together.

Emilio, of the AIDS Generation, actually began developing this consciousness during our interview:

> It's really interesting because I used to be bilingual when I was a kid. And my God. You just made me think of something . . . when the gay thing came up, I kind of stopped speaking Spanish. You just made me realize that. So now, like I could understand everything, but I don't—I'm not fluent anymore.

Similarly, Yasar, who is of African descent, said of his ethnic-racial-sexual struggles, "Ghanaians say that being gay is not African." Juan, both Asian and Latino, specifically Mexican, described how his cultural backgrounds complicated his ability to fully realize his life as gay man:

> [In] the Chinese culture you don't talk about sexuality much, it's [actually] something that you don't ever talk about. And like in a sense like that wasn't even—in my vocabulary. Like, being gay—like, that—that wasn't like one of like the things I could be, really. So yeah definitely well, my mom, I knew like wouldn't understand it. And on the Mexican culture, obviously, it's still very like male dominated and you have to like put up a lot of appearances. And my parents, to some extent, broke from that because they were very internationally minded. But at the same time, you can't get rid of those really deeply rooted cultural mannerisms, I guess.

Since their race or ethnicity already makes them more visible targets for discrimination, another reason racial and ethnic minority gay men may have more trouble coming out is that they may also experience heightened levels of discrimination when they disclose their sexual identity.[7] In fact, gay men of color often employ the same type of hypermasculine behavior used to "cover" sexual identity, as discussed in the previous chapter. A person's race and ethnicity, however, cannot be covered, creating greater stressors and ultimately leading to worse health outcomes as a result of multiple minority stressors.[8]

Black LGBTQ youth are also less likely to be involved in gay social activities, indicating less socialization in gay venues. Some research has shown that this socialization in the gay community is protective in terms of risk,[9,10] but it has also been found that higher levels of gay community affiliation are associated with greater risk in regard to sex and drug use.[11,12] The latter finding underscores the belief that gay community norms modeling and emboldening risky choices must be tackled to improve the health of the men in the community. This is all to say that context matters when seeking to understand coming out and health of gay men.

Environment—including residential, social, and sexual—may interact with race, culture, and ethnicity to shape the coming out process of racial and ethnic sexual minority men, and of first-generation sexual minority men born to immigrant parents,[13,14] most of whom reside in neighborhoods that are segregated due to cultural, economic, and political forces. For these children of immigrants, be they Chinese, Ghanaian, Indian, Greek, or any other ethnicity, being on the "down low"—a term I despise—is as prevalent as it is for African American men in the United States. Unfortunately, that term has become racially embedded, as if the behavior only exists in the black community, and it legitimizes and enables covering, preventing some gay men from ever fully realizing their whole selves. That said, black and Hispanic men may be more likely to be on the down low than white men,[15] but such analyses often ignore the role of foreign-born, immigrant, or first-generation status. Just as gay is not gay is not gay, white is not white is not white.

For young gay men who are members of racial and ethnic minority groups in the United States, the coming out process is complicated by experiences of homophobia, heterosexism, and hypermasculinity in these racial and ethnic environments.[16] Case in point: some 60% of black and 60% of Hispanic votes supported Proposition 8,[17] which sought to deny marriage equality to same-sex couples in California. This level of intolerance in black and Hispanic communities may result from the prevalence of non-LGBTQ-affirming religions within those communities, suggesting that this condition has less to do with race and ethnicity than religion.[18] Social class also plays a role, as it does for white men from working-class backgrounds, in which covering is very much a reality shaped by the culture of their economic class. The stigma these men experience perpetuates and exacerbates the health challenges faced as gay men.

The coming out experience is predicated on all of these intersectional identities—race, ethnic background, immigrant experience, and economic class. For white young gay men from families of means, coming out may be the only challenge they have encountered in their short lives. Whether or not this is true, such depiction reinforces the views of some nonwhite gay men who understand their own coming out experiences as more challenging. As noted by Miguel:

> If you grow up in an American household that identifies as white, I feel like you can have a coming out experience that'll be, not only affirming, but even, like, like wanted. Like, some parents actually want their children to be gay because they think that their kids will live, like, some more fabulous lifestyle than they do.

Miguel was clear about the realities and multiple challenges gay men of color must deal with, specifically those not related to being gay, that may not be present in the lives of gay white men. This situation only makes the coming out process for nonwhite gay men harder, as the difficulties in their lives are compounded.

> The simpler your life is, the less problems you have to think about, which is inherent with white people. [They] think that, you know, that racism isn't a problem because, if you grow up, if you grow up in white supremacy, you don't have much to think about. You don't have problems to think about like that. It's just not your concern.

Juan underscores this idea as well, noting, "[It's easier] if you're white in a society that values whiteness, [society] constantly [helps] white people succeed."

Like Miguel, Juan, and Yasar, gay men of color experience numerous hardships related to their racial backgrounds—struggles informed by race, ethnicity, culture, and class, such as economic status or violence in the neighborhoods in which they were raised. These issues serve to further complicate the negotiation of their sexual identities. Still, the challenge of being gay is just one more issue that they need to navigate: One of the other men with whom we spoke indicated, "Most of the experiences that I had happened, or occurred, [were] due to me being black and gay," or as noted by Huang previously, "I'm not just only gay, I have other labels. I'm Asian American . . . I'm male."

These multiple minority identities have been understood as producing psychosocial burdens, but in the words of Juan, they are also a source of resilience and empowerment, creating an ability to expedite the coming out process more effectively:

> I actually think it might be harder for [white gay men] to like reconcile their gay identity in a way because it's just like they're not used to feeling left out. They're not used to feeling stigmatized, depressed.

In a similar vein, Miguel explained:

> *Being marginalized across any boundaries is going to make you hyper self-aware of other people's issues. Like if you have lots of things to worry about, chances are you have a more profound understanding of how to detangle those problems than other people because they don't have to deal with those sorts of issues.*

The great power and truth in Juan's and Miguel's comments speak to the resilience and grit that young men who have faced adversity are forced to develop. Racial and ethnic sexual minority individuals may actually be better equipped with strategies to counter the impact of heterosexist discrimination of their sexual identity because of the other forms of discrimination they have experienced in their lives.[19] And unfortunately, in the gay community, such strategies are sometimes necessary.

RACISM WITHIN THE GAY COMMUNITY

Intersectional identities and racism, both outside and within the gay community, are intimately linked. These social circumstances led Miguel to understand his life experiences as a gay man of color as different from those of a white gay man. In his view, individuals who hold intersectional identities related to a minority race and gender are not bestowed the same advantages as gay white men, especially hypermasculine white men:

> *[If you are White and gay] the opportunities are still sort of limitless—as long as you can pass as white. As white, and male, you know. Once you start to deviate from that, once you start to be a little bit more effeminate, once you start to realize that maybe you're trans, or maybe you're a person of color, and as you start to deviate from that, what white supremacy deems is the normal, your problems become tenfold, triple fold as the more intersections you add. Opportunities abound if you're, if you're a white guy. It doesn't matter if you're gay or straight.*

Miguel's words highlight the experience of many gay men who are not the archetype that adorns the covers of leading gay publications, the Thor-like, physically strong, quintessential white gay man. We all know these men. Many of us have been, or tried to be, these men—and too many of us have been dismissed and rejected by them.

Embedded in the social conditions that not only expect but also promote hypermasculinity and whiteness, gay men are demeaned and subjected to intolerable terms used to describe each other. For example, there are a multitude of types of "queens" almost always related to race, ethnicity, or culture, such as "rice queen," "dairy queen," and "bean queen." (A rice queen is a white gay man who desires Asian men, a dairy queen is Hispanic man who seeks white men, and so forth.) Such slang is ridiculous, absurd, and unacceptable as it only serves to divide the gay community while supporting the racist power structures prevalent throughout larger society—of course the LBTQ community is not immune.

Racism in the gay community is palpable, further tangible evidence of how members of a marginalized group also tend to marginalize others within the group. Straight people sometimes are surprised or confused by this condition, but they fail to understand that the oppressed may also oppress others. I explained this idea in a 2017 *Newark Star Ledger* op-ed.[20] Perhaps as compelling as the editorial, however, was the homophobic and racist comments on the web page in which it was published. One comment posted by "Ray Z" summarizes the hate faced by gay men, particularly gay men of color, and an obvious inability on the part of "Ray Z" to even consider the social circumstances gay men must confront within their own community: "Who cares if the filthy rump riders don't like dark meat."

In the same Top-10 list of things gay men should stop doing in 2018 mentioned in chapter 6, Lamar Dawson placed racism as #8 with a humorous note that addressed the challenge:

> I'm going to write about this topic until I can no longer type or until racism is more dead than Kevin Spacey's career—whichever happens first. While I just love it when I go to a gay bar and see a sea of white gays singing along to Beyoncé's "Formation" and talking about their love for the Jackson 5's nostrils, while the bartender serves every white gay but me, I'd be fine leaving that in 2017. Also, putting "no rice, no curry" on your dating profile is still racist, not a preference. Fix it before 2018.[21]

Reid understands this racism within the gay community all too well, which he began experiencing at the onset of his life as a gay man in Chicago:

> I think after I graduated from college and moved out [from my parents' home] that's when my racial identity started being like a big deal, like, I've been called a chink by some sick bartenders at, like, big [gay] bars in L.A., Chicago, and New York.

Reid shared one specific incidence that was both enlightening and disheartening:

> I had just moved to Chicago and went in [the bar] by myself, and I got a drink or whatever, and I paid with a $20, and he gave me the change back, and I was

pulling it away to leave him a cash tip because that's what everybody does, and I heard him turn around to his other bartender friend and say, "That chink over there didn't leave me any money. Be sure he doesn't get served anymore," which I heard just blatantly loud. And so, I e-mailed the management: "Hey, I went to this establishment. I'm not mad, I will still continue to support you guys, being a small business and because of where I live and work in the area, but I just wanted to let you know that this happened, this was said by this person," and the e-mail response I got back said, "This is a mindset that we have in Chicago. You're gonna have to get over it," essentially.

The comments by the bartender are truly troubling but unfortunately not surprising; more disturbing is the reaction of the management and perpetuation of the status quo.

This type of racism directly informs the coming out process of many gay men. Compounding the feelings of otherness we all have while coming of age in a heterosexual society, as outlined in the previous chapter, our sense of otherness is perpetuated within the gay community itself as it espouses rigid conceptions of body type, physical appearance, sexual role, penis size, and skin tone. If the boxes are not all checked, men who are still trying to find themselves may be ignored, dismissed, or rejected by the community, further complicating the already complex process of coming out. Reid explains:

I think the reason why it took me so long to lose my virginity and jump into the dating scene and whatnot is because I was never desired. I was never desired because, like, the predominant desired gay man is, like, six feet tall or taller. They're usually white. You know, they have abs or big arms. It's a very convoluted, shallow version of what I think people want.

Such rejection is not uncommon, either in person or online. Though interpersonal dynamics in real time, such as at a bar or a club, make it more challenging to ignore, dismiss, or reject someone because of their appearances, this still occurs more so for people of color, who are either sexually objectified or fetishized. Huang vividly portrayed his experiences as an Asian gay man and the challenges he faced not having the physicality of the archetypal gay man in the 1990s—the white Adonis—which in New York City was referred to as a "Chelsea Boy," since Chelsea had become the center of gay life during that decade:

Champs, Twilo, Roxie. I'm not your typical Chelsea boy. Come on, right, is that really—you look at Next *magazine or HX, I mean it's like, it's all this like—It's kind of like in the regular world, it's like you've got the pecking order. You got the entitled, white male and then there's everyone else. You got the blacks, the Latinos; you got all the little groups and the little Asians, too. Well, the same thing in the gay world, you know, I was quick to navigate that. And in my, 18-, or 19-year-old, I was like, yeah. So, I went, you know, in this world, you have to find yourself and you are usually pigeon-holed, or categorized in one way or another, right. "Oh, Asian, G.A.M. [gay Asian male], okay, bottom." It's like they all assume that.*

Still, Huang isn't necessarily immune from the racial biases he has personally experienced and perpetuates the divide:

I know I'm not sexually attracted to Asians. I just am not. And I'm not attracted sexually to black men, normally. I'm not. You know, but have I seen folks who are Asian and black and are hot as hell? I'm like, hot as hell, but does that mean that I'm gonna go run and chase after them? And say, "Hey, be my boyfriend." Probably not. Maybe for a lay, but not—I'm not wired that way.

This objectification or dismissal of gay men of color, embedded within the racism of the community, occurs even more easily today with the ongoing development of new dating and hookup apps. With a simple slide across the screen of any handheld device, someone's profile can be swept into the trash—as Katy Perry sings, "Swish, swish bish." This attitude and approach has become so prevalent that the Apicha Community Health Center, a health center in New York serving the needs of LGBTQ people, issued guidance in the form of a report titled "Using Hook-Up Apps in 2017":[22]

Let's be real, not talking to someone because they are Asian or Black or Latino or Middle Eastern is not a preference, it's racist. And, PLEASE, stop referring to POC [people of color] as food groups, it's disgusting. And, we will probably need to talk about fetishizing people of color or using the word exotic to initiate a conversation. So, what we are really addressing is the underlying issues of white supremacy and anti-black and brown violence that continues to show itself ever so blatantly on these hook-up apps.

Using such apps, Reid has experienced both racism and sexual objectification as an Asian man by white men—the 21st-century version of Huang's life story:

So [this is] the thing I found most interesting, especially, like, when Grindr and Scruff and all those apps started coming out. I don't consider myself to be the prettiest gay. I'd say I'm relatively put together for the most part. And what I found so interesting is that I was getting even shafted by what we call the rice queens, the guys who are only into Asians, because I didn't fit the stereotypical Asian profile. They wanted me to be 5'6" or less. They wanted me to, like, be a power bottom. They wanted me to speak like I was fresh off the boat.

Reid's and Huang's experiences are unfortunately not unique and may be easily misunderstood or overlooked in the gay community. For example, Daniel Gawthrop wrote an entire memoir, *The Rice Queen Diaries*,[23] in 2005, dedicated to his travels in search of Asian men. While this work is allegedly one of self-discovery and emerging sexuality, it also perpetuates racism within the gay community veiled under sociosexual politics. Moreover the book raises underlying issues with such attractions, as noted by writer Alexander Chee in his 2017 editorial:[24] "I tried to imagine it. Having an erotic imagination so focused on one race of people. All that my ex-boyfriends had in common was me." Chee's words are indicative of the sexual objectification or dismissal of gay men who are not White. In the end, at its core, these attractions or repulsions are at the heart of racism within the gay community.

In this regard, Yasar, a black man, also spoke of experiences akin to those of Reid while using dating and sex apps:

I feel like when it comes to social media, when it comes to like Grindr and stuff like that, there are so many assumptions like the big black guy, like you only do X, Y, and Z. Like you only do one thing or top.

This stereotyping has very much been a part of Yasar's life. While his physicality predisposes hypermasculinity, it in fact is counter to his complex and nuanced understanding and experiences as a man of color who is also gender fluid. Yasar spoke about situations that were emblematic of the racism he has found within the gay community, perpetuated by nonblack men:

You know how nonblack people see black people as far as attractiveness in the queer community. It can range from not being attracted because you're black or because you're dark-skinned. It has some colorism aspects to that. And then your blackness being only for supply—only for, okay so like the BBC thing. I didn't hear that—that big black cock term, I didn't hear that until I came to New York, I was like what is that?

This compartmentalization of black men is rooted in the same social conditions as the typecasting that occurs with Asian men in the gay community. Such racially based "ghettoization" is perhaps more hurtful than out-and-out racist comments, those that are sometimes said in public, but are often more likely made in private. Yasar addressed these types of micro- and macroaggressions:

> It's stereotyping. Yeah, so I feel like that's anti-Black. Because you see a big black guy and you associate that with one thing. And as far as like attractiveness goes within the community as far as like other things. I haven't gotten like a blatant like, "You're not beautiful." Or I guess it's not PC to do the whole like "no blacks, no"— on like Grindr and stuff like that. But people still do it.

These conditions should give serious pause about the amount of work that has to be done to increase awareness around matters of race in our own population of gay men, especially when even those who are aware of the condition maintain racial biases and make racist statements, whether knowingly or not. Some argue that racial preferences by Asian and black men within the community are different than those held by gay white men, as noted by Donovan Trott in a 2017 piece for *The Huffington Post*,[25] "An Open Letter to Gay, White Men: No You Are Not Allowed to Have Racial Preference." In this article, Trott poses the evocative point that racial selection and segregation by men of color may not be racist as it is for white men because of the place of men of color in society.

An interesting thought, though it can also be argued that no matter the source of racist attitudes and preferences, they still need to be scrutinized and condemned if we as a community are to continue progressing together. All gay men should be held to the same standards of civility and discourse and give the respect that is due to each other, else we further perpetuate the underlying toxic issues of racism that plague our community and society as a whole. In approaching this sensitive subject, journalist Frank Bruni wrote an editorial in August 2017, titled "I Am a White Man. Hear Me Out,"[26] in which he eloquently argues that while he is a white man of means, he is also a gay man who has been subjected to the slurs and discrimination of all other gay men. While he recognizes that gay men of color may experience more minority stressors, he also argues that the voice of white gay men cannot be diminished as lesser, stating, "The legitimacy of my voice shouldn't depend on my oppression." He went on to write, "It used to be when someone called me an abomination, I was in the presence of a homophobe. But a recent opinion column damned me for a different reason. I'm abominable because I'm White."

This statement was not meant to dismiss the issues gay men of color must combat every day, especially black and Asian men, often perpetrated by white gay men. The article meant to demonstrate the layers and complexity of intersectionality and racism with the gay population. It is too simple to assume every white gay man is racist and that every gay man of color is not. Instead what is likely true is that years of oppression of communities of color within society, coupled with the fetishizing and/or dismissal of men of color, have led to today's divisions. Bruni's piece was met with mixed reviews.

As a result of these social circumstances, dating and establishing sexual and intimate relationships across race and ethnicity is a complex and complicated situation in the gay community. In some instances, this difficulty manifests in a form of sexual segregation referred to as "sexual racism" by the Apicha Community Health Center— white men choose white men, black men choose black men. Such racial matching aligns with findings about gay men, race, and ethnicity, which were often shown as critical factors to the success of Internet-mediated sexual encounters. In this qualitative study, titled "Internet Sex Ads for MSM and Partner Selection Criteria: The Potency of Race/Ethnicity Online,"[27] gay men of color reported racialized interactions that "ranged from simple expressions of race-based preferences, to blatantly discriminatory or hostile interactions, and often demeaning race-based sexual objectification."

In one study, black men reported higher rates of same-race partners than might be expected solely by chance,[28] which is the likely factor explaining HIV prevalence in younger black gay men. In an attempt to explain this epidemiological pattern as not being due to promiscuity but rather racial homophily—the tendency of individuals from one group to interact and develop relationships solely with people from the same group—an unforeseen byproduct has been the further alienation of gay black men from gay men of other races due to the ongoing stigma and fear of HIV within the gay community. While the data certainly support the notion that a lack of virus management may be at play in perpetuating HIV in young black gay men, it also diminishes black men's desirability as sexual and love partners in the gay community. Unfortunately, in the minds of some gay men, this sexual segregation is justified, as is noted in the words of "Alegoff," who also commented on my *Newark Star Ledger* editorial and sought to justify that "nonattraction" as not racist:

> That being said, it is not racist to not be attracted to everyone. Attraction is not a choice whether it comes to the broader context (straight, gay, bi etc.) or the individual context (specific person) and it is entirely possible for an individual to not be sexually attracted to members of another specific race and not be a racist.

"Alegoff" and others must deeply consider why such an attraction isn't present. Is it due to an inability to look beyond the surface at the many gifts an individual may possess? Or is attraction only skin deep? It seems that the latter opinion or feeling dominates many of the interactions between gay men. Of course, gay men do not reject each other simply because of race but also height, weight, six-pack abs, and hair, to name just a few physical attributes, let alone HIV status.

In light of these realities, it is incredibly important for every gay man who experiences racism within their community to call it out, much as the #MeToo movement has been empowering women to speak out about sexual harassment and assault, no matter if detractors minimize some of the women's claims. We must enact similar approaches with regard to racism in the gay community, calling out every single instance. As noted by historian Ibram Kendi,[29] "the heartbeat of racism is denial." The culture will not change unless we allow the pendulum to swing in the opposite direction and achieve an extreme, before settling somewhere in the middle. Calling out racism, saying it aloud, and announcing the wrong will create a real phenomenon that will effect change, while also fostering safer and more favorable conditions for gay men of color to come out. If these men are embraced by a community, rather than belittled, vilified, or objectified, they will be more comfortable and willing to come out. Instead, the conditions today create stress for young gay men of color who may already be subjected to the intolerance of the sexuality in their families, only to find themselves judged solely on their race or ethnic background in the gay community as well.

TALKING ABOUT RACE AND ETHNICITY ACROSS GENERATIONS

Consciousness and awareness of intersectionality and racism are more highly evident in the coming out stories and life experiences of younger men than their older counterparts. This statement is not a judgment, simply a fact. Throughout the interviews, narratives and dialogue around racism were nearly absent from the conversations with the men of the Stonewall Generation—aside from Wilson, who spoke openly about the racism he encountered as a black gay man coming of age in the 1950s—and only slightly evident in the narratives of the AIDS Generation.

Wilson's racial and sexual narrative was shaped by the time he was born, so he was forced into developing a more nuanced understanding of racism, and the burden it created throughout his life. In fact he experienced more discrimination for his skin tone than his sexual identity while at Harvard:

The gay thing was fine, but the racism, it's a little problematic. I can't say that I had a lot of bad encounters you know, because, I was fortunate enough to meet—I was with university people, and they're usually different in terms of their thinking. You know? So most of the time, the people I was with were educated, and not showing racism. You know? But you had to encounter the store shopkeepers, and the people in the street, the landladies, you know, and the market people. You know? You do encounter that. And I did feel it, you know, the racism. The gay thing was completely different, as I was saying. It was very liberated.

During our interviews, the men of the AIDS Generation addressed issues of intersectionality, but these comments were often made in passing and lacked the depth and passion that emerged from the men of the Queer Generation. Members of my generation were most passionate when they spoke of AIDS, which isn't surprising, considering the evolution of gay rights over the last 50 years and the challenges that shaped each generation.

As members of the AIDS Generation had come out and just begun to secure their place in the world in the 1970s and 1980s, this horrific disease undermined so much of the progress that had been made. The endless, debilitating battle against AIDS continues. Perhaps with the advances in this battle, however, and our rights emerging further within society, an ability to more fully explore what it means to be gay men along aspects of class, race, ethnicity, culture, and class will begin to develop—a product of our previous efforts and the natural evolution of gay rights. This in turn will allow the community to truly embrace the many colors of the rainbow, accepting all colors, shapes, and sizes and challenging the white hypermasculine archetype that is held in such high esteem—an improved community in which it will be easier for all gay men to come out.

As a consciousness of otherness begins to emerge, especially with the Queer Generation, and the fight against marginalization within American society continues by people of color, immigrants, women, and sexual and gender minorities, the gay community must recognize that we also need to be highly conscious of the otherness we perpetuate within our own populations. A fuller understanding must be developed so that the oppressions in our microcosm no longer fuel the condition of society at large. We must reflect within our selves and make changes at the grassroots level within our own communities.

Members of the Queer Generation possess less rigid conceptions of masculinity, more gender and sexual fluidity, and a heightened desire to differentiate themselves from the heterosexual population. They also have a deeper understanding of how race, ethnicity, and intersectionality on a whole play into the gay experience of young men today—a perception that may be lost on older generations, as Yasar pointed out:

> So I feel like there's a lot of divides within the LGBTQ spectrum and community. Like after you know gay marriage was passed, you know that was a good thing, that was cool um, but I just remember that night I went to a gay bar in Charlotte, one of the more popular gay bars. And we're celebrating that win, and I remember arguing with this gay guy, this gay white man, older guy, about the validity of trans women or the lives of trans women. And especially black trans women. And I was like "Are you fucking kidding me?" I don't think this is really a win for me considering that—I mean yeah, I can marry somebody like another man, but again my trans sisters are being killed and they're homeless and they're getting into sex work.

There is a burgeoning recognition that we must attend to the matters of diversity within our population and to the intersectional identities that we hold. In recent years, Pride celebrations throughout the country—in cities like New York; Washington, DC; Columbus, Ohio; and Minneapolis— have been marked by protests seeking to give voice to LGBTQ people of color. At the same time, these protests challenge the corporate infusion into Pride, which mostly celebrates the white gay male experience while ignoring the diversity within the LGBTQ population.[30,31] In 2017, members of the group "No Justice No Pride," a conglomeration of Washington, DC–based activists who challenge the white archetype and marginalization of queer and transgender members of the LGBTQ population, called out the corporate sponsorship, and in turn economic motivation, behind Capital Pride events that exalt the white gay male while marginalizing others in the city's LGBTQ population, including immigrants, the queer, and trans individuals and people of color.[32]

During the same Pride celebration, a redesigned LGBTQ flag was hoisted at a ceremony in Philadelphia.[33] This newer flag, building on the Rainbow Flag first fashioned by the Betsy Ross of the gay movement, Gilbert Baker, incorporates a brown and black stripe above the rest of the rainbow as a symbol of people of color who are often overlooked in the LGBTQ movement and the discrimination evident in our population and the communities we have formed.

FINAL THOUGHTS

Due to America's unfortunate and troubling history, race, ethnicity, culture, and class are complex constructs in America. Today's political climate has only served to polarize the US population even more. The gay population is not immune from these circumstances. Too often we perpetuate the conditions of society at large, targeting men of color as objects of fetishized desires or dismissing them through racial profiling. Many who seek to challenge these racist ways are also silenced. These conditions further complicate the coming out process for men of color. Perhaps this is the reason so many more black and Hispanic men are on the down low—their sexuality is not welcome in their ethnic and racial communities and they are treated as lesser in their sexual community as well.

Though symbolically important, adding a brown and black stripe to the Rainbow Flag is not the solution. The gay population has the opportunity to serve as a model for society at large. Gay men are not the enemy to the queer population. White gay men are not the enemy to gay men of color. The solution is to collectively recognize the enormous diversity that exists within the LGBTQ population and to celebrate and honor it. We cannot move forward as a community if we seek to muffle each other's voices or if we attack each other.

We must recognize the fragility of our rights that we have won over time. Moreover, we must not forget our history, namely the efforts of the Stonewall Generation to love openly and of the AIDS Generation to defeat the physical, emotional, and social ravages of the viral epidemic. The battles and the advances of the past have led us to engage in the current dialogues today about intersectionality, gender, race, and culture. But we need more than discussions, we need to put in the work to become a community that respects our diversity and seeks to ameliorate the undue stressors that people of color and queer people experience. As the Queer Generation leads these efforts, it's imperative to remain aware that if we do not collectively support the lives of the totality of the LGBTQ community, and we create division within our own population, those who truly hate us will use this division as an opportunity to chip away at the progress we have made over the last 50 years. We are all in this together, and we must unite to overcome the obstacles we encounter everyday, both from the outside and from within.

REFERENCES

1. Cole ER. Intersectionality and research in psychology. *Am Psychol.* 2009;64(3):170–180.
2. Jerkins M. Why do you say you're black? *New York Times* 2018.
3. Purdie-Vaughns V, Eibach RP. Intersectional invisibility: the distinctive advantages and disadvantages of multiple subordinate-group identities. *Sex Roles.* 2008;59(5–6):377–391.
4. Hannah D. My struggle to take anti-H.I.V. medicine. *New York Times* 2017.
5. Rosario M, Schrimshaw EW, Hunter J, Braun L. Sexual identity development among gay, lesbian, and bisexual youths: consistency and change over time. *J Sex Res.* 2006;43(1):46–58.

6. Morales ES. Ethnic minority families and minority gays and lesbians. *Marriage Fam Rev.* 1989;14(3–4):217–239.

7. Velez BL, Watson LB, Cox R Jr, Flores MJ. Minority stress and racial or ethnic minority status: a test of the greater risk perspective. *Psychol Sex Orientat Gend Divers.* 2017;4(3):257.

8. Meyer IH. Prejudice, social stress, and mental health in lesbian, gay, and bisexual populations: conceptual issues and research evidence. *Psychol Bull.* 2003;129(5):674–697.

9. Frye V, Koblin B, Chin J, et al. Neighborhood-level correlates of consistent condom use among men who have sex with men: a multi-level analysis. *AIDS Behav.* 2010;14(4):974–985.

10. Mills TC, Stall R, Pollack L, et al. Health-related characteristics of men who have sex with men: a comparison of those living in "gay ghettos" with those living elsewhere. *Am J Public Health.* 2001;91(6):980–983.

11. Green AI, Halkitis PN. Crystal methamphetamine and sexual sociality in an urban gay sub-culture: an elective affinity. *Cult Health Sex.* 2006;8(4):317–333.

12. Halkitis PN, Kapadia F, Siconolfi DE, et al. Individual, psychosocial, and social correlates of unprotected anal intercourse in a new generation of young men who have sex with men in New York City. *Am J Public Health.* 2013;103(5):889–895.

13. Hom AY. Stories from the homefront: perspectives of Asian American parents with lesbian daughters and gay sons. *Amerasia J.* 1994;20(1):19–32.

14. Tremble B, Schneider M, Appathurai C. Growing up gay or lesbian in a multicultural context. *J Homosex.* 1989;17(3–4):253–267.

15. Wolitski RJ, Jones KT, Wasserman JL, Smith JC. Self-identification as "down low" among men who have sex with men (MSM) from 12 US cities. *AIDS Behav.* 2006;10(5):519–529.

16. Brown E. We wear the mask: African American contemporary gay male identities. *J Afr Am Stud.* 2005;9(2):29–38.

17. Coates T-N. Prop 8 and blaming the blacks. *The Atlantic* 2009.

18. Barnes DM, Meyer IH. Religious affiliation, internalized homophobia, and mental health in lesbians, gay men, and bisexuals. *Am J Orthopsychiatry.* 2012;82(4):505–515.

19. Moradi B, Wiseman MC, DeBlaere C, et al. LGB of color and white individuals' perceptions of heterosexist stigma, internalized homophobia, and outness: comparisons of levels and links. *The Counseling Psychologist.* 2010;38(3):397–424.

20. Halkitis PN. Rutgers dean: why racism must be addressed within gay population | Opinion. *Newark Star Ledger* 2017.

21. Dawson L. 10 things gay men should stop doing in 2018. *Logo New Now Next* 2017.

22. Apicha Community Health Center. Using hook-up apps in 2017: emotional health. 2017.

23. Gawthrop D. *The rice queen diaries.* Vancouver: Arsenal Pulp Press; 2009.

24. Chee A. My first (and last) time dating a rice queen. *The Stranger* 2017.

25. Trott D. An open letter to gay, white men: no, you're not allowed to have a racial preference. *Huffington Post* 2017.

26. Bruni F. I'm a white man. Hear me out. *New York Times* 2017.

27. Paul JP, Ayala G, Choi KH. Internet sex ads for MSM and partner selection criteria: the potency of race/ethnicity online. *J Sex Res.* 2010;47(6):528–538.

28. Raymond HF, McFarland W. Racial mixing and HIV risk among men who have sex with men. *AIDS Behav.* 2009;13(4):630–637.

29. Kendi IX. The heartbeat of racism is denial. *New York Times* 2018.

30. Hajela D. Pride and prejudice? Race tinges LGBT celebrations. *AP News* 2017.

31. Arana G. White gay men are hindering our progress as a queer community. *Them* 2017.

32. Stein P, Bui L. Capital Pride parade disrupted by protesters; revelers rerouted. *Washington Post* 2017.

33. Coleman N. Redesigned pride flag recognizes LGBT people of color. *CNN* 2017.

CHAPTER 8

Party and Play

The use of alcohol, tobacco, and other drugs is as old as time in the gay male population and has come to be considered a health disparity in the lesbian, gay, bisexual, transgender, and queer (LGBTQ) population.[1] During the onset of the AIDS epidemic in the United States, substance use, particularly injection drug use, was implicated as a vector for transmission of the virus. Since that time, non-injection drug use has been implicated in the transmission of HIV alongside injection drug use.[2-5] Tellingly, even though gay men use noninjection drugs more than intravenous ones,[6] these drugs are comparable in perpetuating HIV transmission in the gay male population.[7]

Researchers[8,9] documented the use of drugs in the community even before the epidemic took hold. The AIDS crisis, however, illuminated these behaviors, and the most hypersexualizing drug of all, crystal meth, entered the spotlight. Though different forms of methamphetamine (meth) had been used and abused in the United States since the 1950s[10] it wasn't until the 1990s that it began to garner so much attention.

For many gay men, coming of age is tied to using all types of drugs, including alcohol and tobacco. As discussed, in the days before hookup apps, we socialized more frequently in bars and clubs, where we would meet friends and sexual partners, where we could be ourselves—where we could be gay. That said, even in the app era, substance use and abuse remains high among young men emerging into adulthood. This fact is apparent in the P18 Cohort Study[11] that I have been conducting since 2009. In this study, funded by the National Institute on Drug Abuse, we have been following drug use and other health behaviors of a cohort of gay men since they were 18 years old—members of the Queer Generation—documenting patterns of health. This study has helped expand our understanding of sexual minority health for a new generation of gay men whose life experiences are influenced, but not completely defined, by AIDS.

Among the baseline sample of 18-year-olds included in the study, some 51% reported the use of alcohol to the point of intoxication in the month prior to assessment, on an average of 2 days per month. By age 21, this figure rises to 68% and 3 days per month. Approximately 56% also report the use of marijuana and 21% use other drugs including ecstasy, cocaine, and heroin.

In many ways, partying, and the substance use that normally comes hand in hand with it, is a part of many gay men's lives, especially with younger men when they first come out and begin to learn more about themselves. As depicted in both the American and British versions of the television series *Queer as Folk*, alcohol and other drug use is at the heart of these men's experiences as they navigate the social venues of bars, clubs, and circuit parties—large-scale dance parties similar to raves that have their origins in the gay community. These types of gatherings in which gay men get together and dance to all hours of the morning include the annual Black Party in New York City—named so because of its emphasis on leather—and have a decades-old history originating in the East Village bar, The Saint. Parties, such as the Black Party in New York and White Party in Miami, are strongholds of drug and alcohol use among gay men, Bacchanalian feasts of sorts, which are explored in depth in the 2007 book *A Select Body: The Gay Dance Party Subculture and the HIV-AIDS Pandemic.*[12]

Of course many members of the heterosexual population also rely on substances, but the cultural connection between drugs and sexuality in the gay community is much more powerful and prevalent. Tom, who did not use substances until later in his adult life clearly described the link between drugs and social-sexual venues:

> I never did drugs until I was 40 years old. The first experience I had was doing ecstasy and Special K on the dance floor at the Roxy [a dance club], you know. That started a relationship with drugs for me that was primarily a social, you know, going out dancing kind of thing. I got into trouble for a little while with cocaine. I managed to pull myself [out]—it wasn't that long, but it was not good. It was not good. And now, I basically don't do anything although I miss being on a dance floor, with ecstasy. I went to Fire Island this year. I did do it once [while there]. It was kind of like, "Oh, this is what it was like." So, if I were 19, I mean, I would do a lot more of them.

The connection between drug use and gay sexualized social venues is clear in Tom's words, as is his understanding that drug use is very much part of gay culture, especially for younger men. His sentiments also mirror the patterns of drug use across the different generations. During the interviews conducted for this book, the men of the Stonewall Generation rarely talked about drinking or doing drugs, which were nearly absent from their life stories; and it if did evolve it was at an older age as is Tom's life. The men of the AIDS Generation and Queer Generation, however, frequently discussed the role that drugs played in their lives.

The reliance on drugs for some men at the onset of their gay lives can become a lifelong reality, which can lead to elevated mental health disorders—including further substance abuse.[13] In addition, substance use and abuse is also fueled by the norms that are espoused by the gay community.[14] As noted, there is a tight connection between drug use behaviors and sex among gay men, coined as "party and play" (PNP) and "chemsex." The latter term captures the impact of drugs such as crystal meth in driving sexual risk,[15] although drugs like alcohol and marijuana are as influential in undermining sexual safety[16] across all generations.

The use of drugs by members of the LGBTQ population, including gay men, is deeply tied to the stress and victimization they experience over their gay identity[17] and an ongoing antigay bias.[18] These concepts are central to the tenets of minority stress theory,[19] which indicates that the stress gay men experience due to their sexual identity is further compounded by minority stress if they are men of color. Such stress also includes that which is associated with coming out both in greater society and within the gay community. It's not unusual for younger men to first turn to substance use to help handle the stress over their sexual identity and coming out and then continue to use drugs to ease their anxieties in a new community, as noted by one member of the Queer Generation interviewed: "There is that whole issue and then there was when I would go out to gay clubs, I really felt like I needed to drink, um, in order to have fun at these places."

DRUG USE ACROSS GENERATIONS

Throughout history, drugs have been used, and abused, for many purposes, including as a means of coping with life's stress. For gay men, these stressors include the stigma associated with being gay, emanating from family, friends, and society at large. For a large population of gay men, these life stressors also derive from the AIDS epidemic, which has defined our lives for close to four decades. In fact, early in the epidemic, James L. Martin—a pioneer researcher of HIV and gay men's health—and his colleagues[9] documented the close association between drug use and coping with HIV. This association was elaborated on in the tenets of the cognitive escape model, which supports the idea that drugs are used as a mean of dealing with the stressors experienced by gay men, including AIDS.[20] These tenets certainly align with Emilio's understanding of his own drug use:

> The drugs thing for me was more about escape from HIV. And like in the early HIV epidemic, I mean—it gave you energy. It made you feel powerful. It kind of like almost reversed the HIV thing.

Emilio's words point to an interesting aspect regarding the associations between drug use and HIV. Much of the literature on the subject is rooted in the idea that drug use *precedes* HIV and serves as a facilitator of the disease. LGBTQ activist Peter Staley's 2004 New York City–based crystal meth poster campaign that declared "Buy Crystal, Get HIV for Free," and the crusade that followed,[21] was very much in line with this conception. Indeed there is a powerful association between drug use and risky sex, but drugs are also used as a way to deal with the stressors of HIV *after* contracting the virus, which was the case for Staley's crystal use himself when he was younger. In a 2017 study, it was determined that for many meth users, initiation of the drug followed seroconversion as a means of coping with being HIV-positive.[22]

The impetus behind cognitive escape can also be applied to understand the many other stressors gay men experience as a result of simply being gay in a heterosexist world, regular targets of bigotry and discrimination. Whether micro- or macroaggressions, it has been clearly demonstrated that homophobia leads to heightened mental health burdens for gay men.[23] Gay-related stigma as a driver of depression has also been noted in gay men, including gay men of color in the United States.[24] In effect, alcohol and drugs provide an escape from these circumstances—societal hate and judgment—that too often lead to the deterioration of one's self-worth.

Miguel, part of the Queer Generation, started using drugs during his early adolescence as a way to feel better about his sexuality and the bullying he encountered:

> I continued to smoke weed and find alcohol whenever I could around like 13. I wasn't a heavy drinker, but I used to smoke pot a lot. And smoking weed was sort of, like, an ease out of—it was like a self-medicating thing. Just to drown out everything that happened. Everything. The trauma that was associated with being gay, the—I just didn't want to think about those things anymore. I didn't want to think about being picked on that day. I didn't want to think about not fitting in that day or not having any friends. I didn't want to think about anything. So I just wanted to zone out. So I did that every night on, like, my parents' rooftop. I just, like, snuck out the window, smoked weed, crawled back into bed, prayed for a better day tomorrow.

Yasar had a similar experience, but he also got drunk to mask negative feelings associated with his sexuality in fear of rejection from members of his social circles, including his family. Alcohol served as a numbing agent:

> This was, starting off with second semester of sophomore year of college. I was going through a phase where I was drinking a lot, but not as much as later on which I guess we'll get to, because I was just getting fed up with living a lie.

Drugs also provide a cognitive escape for 19-year-old university student Juan:

> I think it takes a lot of insecurities away like being self-conscious. Like I just think about a lot of things, all the time, like my sexuality, like my racial identity, like my studies. And it's [drug use] just an outlet. Like an easy way to just like suppress that and have fun.

No one wakes up one morning and decides to be an alcoholic or a meth addict, nor does drug use happen within isolation, separate from the surrounding context. Rather, life circumstances and the perpetuation of stressful, unmanaged conditions—such as the hate so many gay men experience from friends, family, political and religious leaders, and colleagues, among others—function as stressors, undermining mental health. Psychiatry professor Richard A. Friedman, of Weill Cornell Medical College, eloquently described this idea in his 2017 *New York Times* editorial, "What Cookies and Meth Have in Common." In the piece,[25] Friedman describes how a social environment creates stress and how this stress impacts the brain, making a person susceptible to addiction, whether drugs, food, sex, cigarettes, or any other vice.

As with other drugs, crystal meth releases surges of dopamine, but with meth, the feelings of pleasure are enhanced some 10-times greater than other sensation-producing behaviors, such as eating or having sex.[26] In the absence of effective coping mechanisms, social support, or psychological and psychiatric guidance, drugs dampen negative feelings gay men may have about their sexuality. Many men with whom I spoke during these interviews supported this idea. For example, Emilio, who also saw connections between his drug use and his serostatus, spoke profoundly about the stress created by his socially produced shame over being gay:

> I had shame from the Catholic upbringing. I had shame about being gay. I had shame about HIV/AIDS. I feel the drug use was kinda the way of dealing with that

shame. Because the drug use, when I use drugs, HIV didn't exist. I could just do whatever I wanted. You know, all that kind of sleep with whoever I wanted to. Being gay didn't matter. All that kinda stuff.

Drugs as Norms

Since drugs and alcohol are so prevalent, in part due to the stressors gay men must manage in straight society, their use has been normalized in the gay community. This fact is fully on display any summer night in the haven of Fire Island Pines New York, where gay men ages 18 to 81 make their ways to a series of "T-dances" to drink, do drugs, and seek out sex and love. Such gatherings find their origins in the "High Tea" of British and American Victorian society, which was then coopted and transformed into the Sunday "T-dances" of the pre-Stonewall era. At the time, when homosexuality was still illegal and selling alcohol to gay men was not permitted, gay men would gather in clubs on Fire Island to dance and meet other men. These dances occurred midday, avoiding the raids that many gay bars incurred during the night time when society was fast asleep, but patrons still needed to keep an eye on the ferry schedule to make sure they returned to the mainland in time.[27] Not much has changed in the last five decades on Fire Island—except now the party takes place from dusk to dawn.

The gay community itself plays a critical part in perpetuating alcohol and drug use, informed by two conditions. First, alcohol and drug use by gay men both within and outside social venues has become normalized. Second, the judgment of gay men's physical appearance by other gay men—as discussed in chapters 6 and 7—lead to a diminished self-worth, exacerbating the negative feelings created by society at large. Lorenzo, a member of the AIDS Generation, addressed both of these issues as he described his desire to fit in with the gay men at a bar in Long Island, New York, that he frequented. He wanted to be with, and like, the men he met there—a desire that may have fueled his drug use at a young age when he was first coming out:

The substance abuse, it was, again, fitting in. I don't know if it was—I'm gonna chalk it up to not being addicted to it. It was more about fitting in because, you know, here I was, coming out. And I came out, and I'm out with these guys. And as far as I can see, they were the "A" crowd. They were the clique to be seen with. So, whatever they did, I did. I went along with it. And in my mind, "Ah, it's only coke. It's not—you know, it's not hallucinogens, it's not PCP, it's not heroin. I'm not gonna shoot a needle in my arm. It's only blow. I can deal with it."

Seth, another member of the AIDS Generation, who was a professional dancer in his younger life, was also introduced to drugs through the gay community around him:

> Paul was a deejay, is a deejay, so he became a bridge, into a completely different world. It was like this re-introduction to the dance world, dance life, dance culture, dance drugs, parties, whatnot, and for me it became all of that and just an entire world of new music. I mean, I had not experienced club music before, not like that, and we were part of the big fan and flag community. It felt like a family and it was alive and very fairy and free, and I was in—again. It felt like I was in a candy store and even though I had this steady relationship, I was as sexual and playful as could be.

Seth had a desire to fit in and be part of what was undoubtedly an exclusive environment, a stronghold of gay elites akin to Lorenzo's "A-list." By modeling drug use for each other, the environments in which we socialize engender drug and sex risk.[28-30] The drive to be desirable within certain parts of the gay subculture then perpetuates the use of drugs, such as crystal meth.[31] Community plays a critical role in both normalizing substances, including tobacco, and sexual risk. These behaviors are also more highly evident among young gay men with stricter ties to the gay community.[32,33] As a result, for some people, like Huang, there is a recognition that they must disengage from many gay social venues in order to avoid succumbing to these pressures:

> I saw a lot of friends who were doing like hard stuff: meth, cocaine, like run of the mill crazy shit. And I stayed away, I was like, "Hmm, I can't." So, like my initial group of friends, back in my early years, you know, the [gay dance clubs] Twilo and the Roxie, it was like, that was what everyone did. You kind of like dropped your E and you'd drink your water, and you'd have a good time. You know, I tried it. It's just not me. So, I was smart. I was smart enough to, like, break away from that group who kept on partying and partying, and partying, and partying, and partying. And I was kind of like, "I need to find myself another group." And I went to sports leagues. And found myself at Gotham volleyball. And everyone there in that specific group, you know, wasn't into the bar scene, wasn't into the drug stuff at all. It was very much—various ages—and we had one thing in common, yes, it was the volleyball that brought us together, but it was definitely, you know, I felt very safe and happy that I was able to escape all that drug shit.

Huang's words and actions must be emphasized, as it would be overly simplistic to think of every gay man as a drug user, although some haters espouse such a notion. In fact, most gay men do not do drugs. Still, depictions of gay life often focus on this aspect. I have long argued, and have for the most part shown across many of my studies, that for every ~20% of gay men who don't use condoms, ~80% do; so too for the ~30% of gay men who use drugs, ~70% do not. In a recent survey study of gay and bisexual men,[34] about one-third of a 3,000-person sample indicated "no drug use" in the 6 months prior to assessment, and therefore did not partake in chemsex.

Such findings are relatively consistent across studies, debunking the myth that all gay men are drug-using sexual addicts parading in the nude during Gay Pride, albeit this stereotypical image is too often depicted in the mainstream media. More importantly, these findings point to the development of health programs and drug use prevention strategies based on resiliencies rather than deficit.[35,36] Such an approach to health programming should be directed by what so many gay men are doing right versus what they are doing wrong.

Like Huang, Lorenzo, relying on his determination and grit, was able to remove himself from social conditions that fueled drug use. Unfortunately, this positive life change also resulted in the loss of his close friends:

> And I couldn't deal with it because, um, there was a point where it got out of control. But I was able—I was strong enough to just go, "That's it. I'm out." And I literally walked away from that entire world. I missed a lot of the people. I'm not gonna demonize them or make them criminals. They're just people doing what they did. And to this day, I've never judged. And I miss them a lot.

Masculinity and Drug Use

Drug use within the male gay community is further informed by the expectations we too often place on each other with regard to our physicality, often our masculinity, as touched on in chapter 6. University of New South Wales professor Garret Prestage and his colleagues[34] have documented the adverse effects of masculine conceptions on the well-being of gay men, particularly as a driver of sexualized drug use (aka PNP and chemsex). Hypermasculine expectations create vulnerability—another point of stress—as gay men seek to achieve a physical ideal within their community. Not living up to this ideal often triggers feelings of otherness for those who do not adhere to archetypes of gay white manliness and who, in turn, are either ignored or fetishized. The expectation of hypermasculinity has been associated with diminished mental health in gay men as they strive endlessly to achieve this physical ideal.[37] Given these social expectations, it's no surprise that some gay men turn to drugs, such as crystal meth, to ease their social engagement, especially when first entering the community after coming out.[38]

Reid, a member of the Queer Generation in his late 20s, clearly understands these conditions dominating gay life in some circles, leading him to rely on drugs as a social crutch:

> I lose any inhibitions. I don't feel like I need to act a certain way or do a certain thing, but—I think that [is what it] boils down to. There are standards in the gay community and we feel we have to adhere to said standards, and if you break away from that, then you're looked at as weird or an outsider in the gay community.

Similarly for Juan, alcohol provided a means of social lubrication, especially early in his development as a gay man:

> I think at the beginning when I was starting to do things with guys, I had to drink to allow myself to justify it and—and yeah, it just makes me more confident, I guess. I think it—it definitely helps like the interaction and makes it; it makes me like less nervous.

As a result of such social conditions within the gay community, the use of substances—especially hypersexualizing drugs such as methamphetamine—lessen social inhibition, enhance self-perception, and heighten sexual activity.[39] The desire for sexual pleasure likely precipitates the use of drugs as they diminish inhibition and enhance a feeling of self-worth, at least in the short term.[40,41] The rigid norms within the gay population exacerbate the burdens created by society more generally and fuel sexualized drug use. Efforts to address drug use in our community must attend to the normalization of these behaviors and the unrealistic expectations we place on each other in terms of our physical and sexual prowess. If not, we will never be able to provide the necessary support for each other and those of us looking for a safe space in which to come out and be comfortable in our own skin.

HEALTH CONSEQUENCES OF PNP

For many gay men, the use of alcohol and other drugs is directly connected to their sexuality and sexual activity. The meth-sex link, the alcohol-sex link, the cocaine-sex link, the "whatever drug it is"–sex link has defined so many of our lives and, in turn, has given the false impression to young people coming of age and developing their sexual identity that drug use is simply part of the LGBTQ culture. Drugs are so evident in our sexual lives that early reports of HIV attributed the disease to the use of inhalant nitrates (poppers). While poppers are not directly the cause of HIV, their use during the sexual acts that transmitted HIV implicated the substance as a culprit. Today this ubiquitous substance—very popular during my generation—continues to be widely used and is highly related to sexual risk.[42] Ultimately, drug use creates challenges for the sexual health of gay men since this mental health burden engenders sexual risk.[43] It is for this reason that PNP has garnered so much attention in the last several decades.

In a similar vein, recreational Viagra use is also implicated in the ongoing transmission of HIV,[44] though, like poppers, not directly. Taking Viagra allows men to have sex for extended periods of time, and across many partners, as it counters the erectile dysfunction created by stimulants such as crystal meth. In our 2005 BUMPS study, another investigation funded by the National Institute on Drug Abuse, in which we followed and documented club drug use and sex risk in a cohort of 450 gay men, some 50% of men reported combining Viagra with methamphetamines.[30] If this all sounds like a culture of "sex, drugs, and rock and roll," that is because drug use among gay men is very much understood as part of a particular lifestyle.

Drug Use for Sexual Lubrication

Sociologist Isaiah Green and I examined this phenomenon with regard to methamphetamine use among New York City–based gay men.[31] We found that though individual factors such as self-esteem and social awkwardness are related to the use of meth, the social pressure of peak sexual performance within the Manhattan gay sexual subculture heightens and exacerbates them. Since methamphetamines are associated with increased self-esteem, libido, and sexual endurance, along with diminished sexual inhibition and a higher threshold for pain, such stimulants are strategically employed to negotiate sexual social situations and increase sexual pleasure.

In this regard, Stephanos, of the AIDS Generation, has used drugs in the search for, and enjoyment of, both sex and love. Describing his first relationship, Stephanos noted:

> Actually the first time I started doing any heavy drugs, and it was ecstasy, was because it was the only time that he ever like would tell me like he loved me. Like, this is like when we were 24. And then I wanted to do ecstasy because I always wanted those—you know those six hours later after the dancing was done and we were back home and like the things he would say to me and the sex was hot.

This desire for love cannot be understated. As we grapple with our sexuality, love provides an affirmation for our identity and our self-worth; it is where we can find the fortitude to combat the negativity of our families and a heterodominant society. In light of these circumstances, it is understandable that Stephanos, in his quest for love, could and would turn to drugs as a means to an end. Moreover, as our identities as gay men are tied very much to sex, Stephanos understands drugs as a mechanism that frees him to have the type of sex that he had always fantasized about.

> We did [coke]—we didn't do it to have sex originally, but it became a big part of sex later. Like—like I realize that it's just like I like—for both of us uninhibiting.

Drug use by gay men is also predicated by the drive for a certain type of fantastical sex, one that seems more remarkable under the influence, in which inhibitions disappear and sense and feelings are heightened. For example, gay men are more likely to engage in esoteric aspects of sex including fisting, feltching, watersports, and other such activities at higher rates when under the influence of crystal meth.[15] This sexually adventurous attitude and fantastical sex undertaken while under the influence of meth creates a psychological dependence on the drug directed more by a type of sex engendered by the drug than the drug itself. Describing such an episode of sexualized drug use, 49-year-old Seth shared the following story around the events of 9/11:

> I remember being in Connecticut on September 11th, fucking my brains out with a guy that I was dating at the time and like, we were in, like, this weekend haze of meth and K and then all of a sudden we turned on—oh yeah, the phone kept ringing, and people are like, "Look at the news, look at the news," then we turned on the news and we're both like, "Holy shit!" and everything said don't drive into New York right now, just stay where you are and we both looked at each other and said, "Okay, let's go fuck." I mean, it's like, there's nothing else to do, um, as long as, you know, once we found out that everybody was safe.

This understanding of drugs' influence on sex, and vice versa, is also very much true to the experiences of young gay men like Miguel:

> Tina, GHB, poppers, cocaine, MDA, all of that shit makes you want to fuck. And straight people, I mean, I don't really know what straight people do to be totally honest. But I know that gay men want to fuck and they'll fuck on anything, within

the right state of mind, you know. Like, I took a bunch of E. I would run through the streets, go to, like, the Eagle or something in Boston, find someone to make out with, have him reach down my pants, you know, it just—the rush, the moment, like, and if anything, men, specifically cis men are very sex driven.

There are cultural, emotional, political, and social dimensions to being gay—those discussed throughout the book—but, at its core, being a gay man is also very much defined by those with whom we have sex, namely other men. Sexual behavior and arousal are part of a person's gay identity development—to deny that the sex we have is not central to who we are would be foolhardy.

The challenge for gay men is that we are not taught how to have sex or love each other. We develop as sexual beings never properly schooled about gay sex. Rather we rely on our own fantasies and imaginations or the imagery presented to us in pornography and other media. For those of us first coming out, gay sex may seem awkward, confusing, and even frightening. The physicality of sex, particularly anal sex, may create challenges for some men. And that's where drugs come back in: they function as a lubricant, both socially, emotionally, and physically, as we clumsily attempt to figure out how to have sex with another man. Drugs like crystal meth facilitate the ability to bottom and manage the potential discomfort associated with this sexual behavior, allowing men to create this physical connection. No sexual interaction will come close to mimicking the perfection of the sex depicted in a pornographic film—let's face it, it's unlikely the repairman will ever be *that* hot—just as no relationship will ever attain the boundless love free of conflict and full of bliss that is the heart and soul of any rom-com. These idealized conditions result in expectations that may be unattainable, creating challenges in our lives akin to those of young girls who grow up only to harshly, and often abruptly, discover that Prince Charming is an imaginary creature that lives solely in fairy tales.

For gay men, these depictions of sex are informed by men of physical perfection, often the hypermasculine, white, archetype, espousing an "ideal man" who is able to have sex for hours on end. In the absence of drugs—including anabolic steroids and PDE-5 inhibitors like Viagra, often used together—this supposedly ideal pornographic sex is a somewhat unattainable reality.[45] The fact is that as gay men we are not taught how to have sex with each other, so some of our early assumptions, fueled by pornography and other media, can turn out wrong. One of my most cherished mentees, Dan Siconolfi, who is now a gay men's health researcher in his own right, and I used to joke that we should write a handbook on the rules of gay sex that would reside on three essential pillars: "shower, shave, and douche."

As mentioned earlier in the book, even in conditions where schools provide sex education, few address same-sex behaviors—instead providing lessons that are useless and meaningless for those of us who are gay. The Gay Lesbian and Straight Education Network[46] found that only about half of LGBTQ students who received sex education found it to be useful, a figure that jumps to 70% for their straight peers. Just like many people I know of my generation, I had the same experience. Fortunately, my very kind and inclusive teacher Mr. Jacobson taught hygiene. While he did not cover the topic of gay sex, he did have guest speakers throughout the class, including one week in which gay men came in to discuss their lives. Hearing these men speak, with my girlfriend sitting next to me—I was still covering at the time—I felt like I was no longer alone in the world or an anomaly. In so many ways, that teacher helped me on my path to fulfilling my sexual identity. It was 1980. Years later I would go back to Bronx High School of Science to be a guest speaker on HIV for Mr. Jacobson's class.

As I was writing this section, my husband, Bobby, was reading over my shoulder and said, "You're right. It wasn't odd kissing a man for the first time. But when we got to the more intimate part, I didn't know if I had to be the top or the bottom or what that meant. And I wasn't ready to bottom. No one told me I had to get ready." Bobby's latter point alludes to the physical realities of men having sex together, aligned with the motto "shower, shave, and douche" that Dan and I would often recite.

Alcohol and drugs provide an escape from the physical challenges of two men having sex—challenges that are bound by biology but also linked to emotions about being gay. As Miguel explained:

> The act of gay sex in itself can be a messy experience. It has a level of cleanliness, and preparation, and things that I think straight people just don't have to worry about. I feel like a lot of men, like, myself included who think about, like, you know, preparation, thinking about going forward with this sort of thing. And with sex, if you, if you do a bunch of Tina and, a bunch of poppers, and some GHB, who gives a fuck if you shit the bed or whatever. Like, they're just gonna keep fucking you. Your mind is lost. It's all gone, and you kind of get to experience a sort of mindlessness. It's all great. Pleasurable and everything's fine, and, like, everything's not fine, but you dupe yourself into thinking that it is.

Miguel's words speak truth. Engaging in anal sex requires preparation and attention. However there is little information out there for gay men, certainly not in high school sex education class, to prepare us for the ins and outs of anal sex, literally and figuratively.

The Mayo Clinic website[47] provides some guidance for men having sex with men, including how to protect oneself from sexually transmitted infections (STIs), tackle depression, address body image concerns, seek help for substance use, and recognize domestic violence. Though the Mayo

Clinic may have meant well, when rephrased, this information implies that gay men are disease-carrying, depressed, body-shaming drug addicts who beat each other up, such a sexy and romantic notion that would send any young gay man negotiating his sexuality running back into the closet.

There is no sex positivity included in this description—no useful information for gay men coming of age to help them understand how their bodies work with one another. Instead, this dispassionate litany of directives is so clinical in its treatment of gay sex that it acts as the other bookend of the equally unhelpful and unrealistic pornographic depictions of gay sex.

Instead of socializing gay men to think about matters of intimacy, passion, and commitment, helping them to prepare to engage with each other physically and in social venues, mainstream society and even some members of the gay community have spent the last four decades berating gay men about condom use and how to avoid acquiring HIV. We have treated gay men as if they are in a relationship with a virus rather than with other men. Human desires for intimacy and passion are squelched when both sex and love are overshadowed by fear and disease prevention. In fact, condoms act as much as emotional barriers as physical ones for gay men, precluding us from achieving connections with another human being when we are constantly on guard against what that individual may transmit to us. Negotiating these feelings and desires, seeking to connect emotionally and physically with another man, is a tall order when the messages about such connections are rooted solely in the avoidance of HIV.

The situation is made all the worse by one book intended for gay men exploring their sexuality, *How to Bottom Like a Porn Star*,[48] based on interviews with members of the porn industry. The book claims to provide a "behind-the-scenes, no-holds-barred look into the industry and the secrets they use to get performers to bottom without pain or messy scenes."

It is no wonder gay men continue to dismiss perfectly wonderful men in their perpetual, futile search for the lover who will provide them a lifetime of awesome passionate sex. Quite frankly, Cosmo's "A Complete Beginner's Guide for Anal Sex"[49] is more informative, despite the fact that it is written for straight women. Fortunately we live in the era of the Internet: one helpful article by Rico Woods on gaypopbuzz.com[50] provides 10 practical, insightful tips for men—who are not porn stars—to physically, emotionally, and socially engage in anal sex. And today, that's what's needed: information spread far and wide to help gay men early in their journey—or even later in their life—to make healthy, positive choices while experiencing the pleasure of sexual activity and connections without fear, confusion, or shame.

It would be misleading of me to not mention the *Joy Of Gay Sex* originally published in 1977 and of great importance to men of the Stonewall

Generation as means of positively affirming sexuality. Still, the need for same sex education must commence during childhood in order to foster the self-acceptance we all need as a gay men. Even though the *Joy of Gay Sex* is beautifully intentioned (and illustrated) its impact may be more limited in enhancing sense of worth or in helping us learn how to relate to each other by the time the volume likely reaches most gay men during their adulthood.

FINAL THOUGHTS

For almost two decades I have studied the complex interplay that exists between substance use and sex in gay men. This scholarship has led me to consider not only the use of particular substances like methamphetamines but also the synergy between drug use, sex risk, and the transmission of HIV and other STIs in the gay male population. This research has also led me to deeply consider why substance use is so rampant in our community, although it is essential to note that *rampant* does not imply the majority, and in fact these behaviors are supported in the minority in most studies.

Drugs provide a momentary reprieve from these issues, a time when men can let their inhibitions go, facilitating sex physically, emotionally, and socially. Drugs also provide a sense of escape for young men coming out, or who want to come out, but are worried about the implications of doing so. Even once these young men do come out, they may face bullying, bigotry, and other discrimination, all of which only further contributes to feelings of the need to escape. On entering the gay community, they may find that drugs are also there to ease their transition into their new lifestyle or help them connect with others.

The emotions associated with sex may also create challenges for gay men as we seek to love and be inmate with each other, despite being raised in a heterosexist world that provides us with no education on how to relate with other men on this level. The social conditions in our community around unreal expectations of physical beauty and perfection only exacerbate the situation. Crystal meth and other similar drugs are therefore used to help facilitate intimacy and emotional connectedness with other men, diminishing our inhibitions and easing our social interactions as we navigate the bars and clubs of days gone by and the e-communities of today.

If we are to truly address this complex drug-sex link, it is insufficient to focus solely on the related behaviors and problems only after young gay men have merged into adulthood. We must start by providing affirming same-sex education in schools that will empower young gay men, who are beginning to make sense of their identities, to love their bodies and to love themselves. Equipped with these self-affirming emotions, the need to escape through drugs and sex will diminish, creating a path for developing fulfilling loving sexual relationships made with open and clear hearts and minds.

REFERENCES

1. Graham R, Berkowitz B, Blum R, et al. *The health of lesbian, gay, bisexual, and transgender people: Building a foundation for better understanding.* Washington, DC: Institute of Medicine; 2011.
2. Halkitis PN, Pollock JA, Pappas MK, et al. Substance use in the MSM population of New York City during the era of HIV/AIDS. *Subst Use Misuse.* 2011;46(2–3):264–273.
3. Stall R, Purcell DW. Intertwining epidemics: a review of research on substance use among men who have sex with men and its connection to the AIDS epidemic. *AIDS Behav.* 2000;4(2):181–192.
4. Ostrow DG, VanRaden MJ, Fox R, Kingsley LA, Dudley J, Kaslow RA. Recreational drug use and sexual behavior change in a cohort of homosexual men. The Multicenter AIDS Cohort Study (MACS). *AIDS.* 1990;4(8):759–765.
5. Rosario M, Schrimshaw EW, Hunter J. A model of sexual risk behaviors among young gay and bisexual men: longitudinal associations of mental health, substance abuse, sexual abuse, and the coming-out process. *AIDS Educ Prev.* 2006;18(5):444–460.
6. Voetsch AC, Lansky A, Drake AJ, et al. Comparison of demographic and behavioral characteristics of men who have sex with men by enrollment venue type in the National HIV Behavioral Surveillance System. *Sex Transm Infect.* 2012;39(3):229–235.
7. Strathdee SA, Stockman JK. Epidemiology of HIV among injecting and non-injecting drug users: current trends and implications for interventions. *Curr HIV/AIDS Rep.* 2010;7(2):99–106.
8. Martin JL. Drug use and unprotected anal intercourse among gay men. *Health Psychol.* 1990;9(4):450–465.
9. Martin JL, Dean L, Garcia M, Hall W. Barbara Snell Dohrenwend memorial lecture. The impact of AIDS on a gay community: changes in sexual behavior, substance use, and mental health. *Am J Community Psychol.* 1989;17(3):269–293.
10. Halkitis PN. *Methamphetamine addiction: Biological foundations, psychological factors, and social consequences.* Washington, DC: American Psychological Association; 2009.
11. Halkitis PN, Cook SH, Ristuccia A, et al. Psychometric analysis of the Life Worries Scale for a new generation of sexual minority men: the P18 Cohort Study. *Health Psychol.* 2018;37(1):89–101.
12. Lewis LA, Ross MW. *A select body: The gay dance party subculture and the HIV/AIDS pandemic* .London, UK: Burns & Oates; 1995.
13. Gilman SE, Cochran SD, Mays VM, Hughes M, Ostrow D, Kessler RC. Risk of psychiatric disorders among individuals reporting same-sex sexual partners in the National Comorbidity Survey. *Am J Public Health.* 2001;91(6):933–939.
14. Carpiano RM, Kelly BC, Easterbrook A, Parsons JT. Community and drug use among gay men: the role of neighborhoods and networks. *J Health Soc Behav.* 2011;52(1):74–90.
15. Halkitis PN, Shrem MT, Martin FW. Sexual behavior patterns of methamphetamine-using gay and bisexual men. *Subst Use Misuse.* 2005;40(5):703–719.

16. Halkitis PN, Bub K, Stults CB, Bates FC, Kapadia F. Latent growth curve modeling of non-injection drug use and condomless sexual behavior from ages 18 to 21 in gay, bisexual, and other YMSM: the P18 Cohort Study. *Subst Use Misuse.* 2018;53(1):101–113.

17. Garnets L, Herek GM, Levy B. Violence and victimization of lesbians and gay men: mental health consequences. *J Interpers Violence.* 1990;5(3):366–383.

18. Cochran SD. Emerging issues in research on lesbians' and gay men's mental health: does sexual orientation really matter? *Am Psychol.* 2001;56(11):931–947.

19. Meyer IH, Frost DM. Minority stress and the health of sexual minorities. In: Patterson C, D'Augelli AR, eds. *Handbook of psychology and sexual orientation.* New York: Oxford University Press; 2013:252–266.

20. McKirnan DJ, Ostrow DG, Hope B. Sex, drugs and escape: a psychological model of HIV-risk sexual behaviours. *AIDS Care.* 1996;8(6):655–669.

21. Fierstein H, Carlson D, Kellerhouse B, Staley P, Tierney S, Lee S. A public forum–challenging the culture of disease: the crystal meth-HIV connection. *J Gay Les Psycho.* 2006;10(3–4):9–43.

22. Halkitis PN, Levy MD, Solomon TM. Temporal relations between methamphetamine use and HIV seroconversion in gay, bisexual, and other men who have sex with men. *J Health Psychol.* 2016;21(1):93–99.

23. Mays VM, Cochran SD. Mental health correlates of perceived discrimination among lesbian, gay, and bisexual adults in the United States. *Am J Public Health.* 2001;91(11):1869–1876.

24. Wohl AR, Galvan FH, Carlos JA, et al. A comparison of MSM stigma, HIV stigma and depression in HIV-positive Latino and African American men who have sex with men (MSM). *AIDS Behav.* 2013;17(4):1454–1464.

25. Friedman RA. What cookies and meth have in common. *New York Times* 2017.

26. Warth G. Kamikaze pilots, Beats and Hells Angels all part of meth crisis history. *North County Times* 2007.

27. Kohler W. The very gay and interesting history of the almost lost tradition of the Sunday tea dance. *Back2Stonewall* 2018.

28. Natale AP. HIV transmission factors: Denver MSM culture and contexts. *J HIV AIDS Soc Serv.* 2008;7(3):241–264.

29. Braine N, Acker CJ, van Sluytman L, Friedman S, Des Jarlais DC. Drug use, community action, and public health: gay men and crystal meth in NYC. *Subst Use Misuse.* 2011;46(4):368–380.

30. Halkitis PN, Green KA, Mourgues P. Longitudinal investigation of methamphetamine use among gay and bisexual men in New York City: findings from Project BUMPS. *J Urban Health.* 2005;82(1 Suppl 1):i18–i25.

31. Green AI, Halkitis PN. Crystal methamphetamine and sexual sociality in an urban gay subculture: an elective affinity. *Cult Health Sex.* 2006;8(4):317–333.

32. Halkitis PN, Kapadia F, Siconolfi DE, et al. Individual, psychosocial, and social correlates of unprotected anal intercourse in a new generation of young men who have sex with men in New York City. *Am J Public Health.* 2013;103(5):889–895.

33. D'Avanzo PA, Halkitis PN, Yu K, Kapadia F. Demographic, mental health, behavioral, and psychosocial factors associated with cigarette smoking status among young men who have sex with men: the P18 Cohort Study. *LGBT Health.* 2016;3(5):379–386.

34. Prestage G, Hammoud M, Jin F, Degenhardt L, Bourne A, Maher L. Mental health, drug use and sexual risk behavior among gay and bisexual men. *Int J Drug Policy.* 2018;55:169–179.

35. Halkitis PN. *The AIDS generation: Stories of survival and resilience.* New York: Oxford University Press; 2013.

36. Halkitis PN, Krause KD, Vieira DL. Mental health, psychosocial challenges and resilience in older adults living with HIV. *HIV and Aging.* 2017;42:187–203.

37. Fischgrund BN, Halkitis PN, Carroll RA. Conceptions of hypermasculinity and mental health states in gay and bisexual men. *Psychol. Men Masc.* 2012;13(2):123.

38. Halkitis PN, Fischgrund BN, Parsons JT. Explanations for methamphetamine use among gay and bisexual men in New York City. *Subst Use Misuse.* 2005;40(9–10):1331–1345.

39. Halkitis PN, Levy MD, Moreira AD, Ferrusi CN. Crystal methamphetamine use and HIV transmission among gay and bisexual men. *Curr Addict Rep.* 2014;1(3):206–213.

40. Cabaj RP. Substance abuse, internalized homophobia, and gay men and lesbians: psycho-dynamic issues and clinical implications. *J Gay Les Psycho.* 2000;3(3–4):5–24.

41. Romanelli F, Smith KM, Pomeroy C. Use of club drugs by HIV-seropositive and HIV-seronegative gay and bisexual men. *Top HIV Med.* 2003;11(1):25–32.

42. Plankey MW, Ostrow DG, Stall R, et al. The relationship between methamphetamine and popper use and risk of HIV seroconversion in the multicenter AIDS cohort study. *J Acquir Immune Defic Syndr.* 2007;45(1):85–92.

43. Batchelder AW, Ehlinger PP, Boroughs MS, et al. Psychological and behavioral moderators of the relationship between trauma severity and HIV transmission risk behavior among MSM with a history of childhood sexual abuse. *J Behav Med.* 2017;40(5):794–802.

44. Fisher DG, Reynolds GL, Ware MR, Napper LE. Methamphetamine and Viagra use: relationship to sexual risk behaviors. *Arch Sex Behav.* 2011;40(2):273–279.

45. Rosen RC, Catania JA, Ehrhardt AA, et al. The Bolger conference on PDE-5 inhibition and HIV risk: implications for health policy and prevention. *J Sex Med.* 2006;3(6):960–975.

46. Human Rights Campaign. A call to action: LGBTQ youth need inclusive sex education. https://www.hrc.org/resources/a-call-to-action-lgbtq-youth-need-inclusive-sex-education. Accessed July 8, 2018.

47. Mayo Clinic Staff. Health issues for gay men and men who have sex with men. 2017. https://www.mayoclinic.org/healthy-lifestyle/adult-health/in-depth/health-issues-for-gay-men/art-20047107. Accessed July 12, 2018.

48. Miller W. *How to bottom like a porn star: The ultimate guide to gay sex* (The How-To Gay Sex Series Book 1). Woodpecker Media; 2014.

49. Breslaw A. A complete beginner's guide to anal sex. *Cosmopolitan* 2017.

50. Woods R. First time bottoming: 10 anal tips for gay men. *Gay Pop Buzz.*

Conclusion

Dignity

The dignity of gay men is intimately linked with our fortitude and grit—our individual and collective resilience. I have come to understand this resilience as both a trait and a dynamic adaptive process, one that includes a temperament allowing us to confront life challenges and develop a feedback loop of actions and coping mechanisms.[1] Resilience is the key component in the lives of all of the men with whom I spoke for this book as they challenged the adversities thrust on them as gay men; it is also at the heart of dignity, whether that dignity be how we conduct ourselves on a daily basis or the lifelong circumstances we navigate in coming out and seeking acceptance from others—and from ourselves.

Despite the conditions that shape our lives from an early age, hurtful and discriminatory acts—some of them state-sanctioned and others simply within our daily routines—run counter to our dignity, perpetuating and exacerbating our feelings of otherness. These conditions can be debilitating, leading to the heightened rates of mental health issues and substance use seen in gay men. But these challenges also function to further bolster our resilience.[2] As former Danish ambassador Rufus Gifford has explained, his sexual identity as a gay man created a discomfort for him in his hometown and forced him to leave this town and take risks in his life. Being gay served as a catalyst for Gifford to summon his grit and fortitude and to make his own place in the world away from his hometown, which parallels my own escape from the shackles of traditional Greek American society in Astoria, Queens, New York, and is a common course of action among many gay men I know and many of those whom I spoke with for this book. Because of the conditions in society, being gay requires we call upon and enhance our resilience.

Dignity is not an attribute that gay men or the lesbian, gay, bisexual, transgender, and queer (LGBTQ) community are given or granted. It has only been earned throughout the course of our lives as we have muddled through constant challenges. Like women and African Americans, the laws of our country were not written for us. The US Constitution was not designed to protect the lives and dignity of LGBTQ people, women, or people of color. The battles in which all of these groups have partaken have been necessary to uncover and own their dignity. These battles manifested in the Stonewall Riots of 1969, the 1913 Suffrage Parade, and the Newark Rebellion of 1967, among many others. And the fight wages on today, as our political rights are challenged by the courts of the land and our lives are cut short through unnecessary killings perpetuated by the vitriol of our American society. Despite the advances in our civil rights, we continue to be placed on the margins and viewed as outsiders to the norm—it remains a dangerous place for all of us.

For those of us who choose to be parents, a wide array of laws and cumbersome processes define who can and cannot be parents, creating legal, social, and emotional challenges for same-sex couples with children.[3] And for LGBTQ people of color the struggle is compounded, as issues of race and racism are experienced within society at large and within the gay community.[4] One of the many challenges for our community is to shift the dialogue of "Pride" back to one that is less about partying, dancing, and white gay male centricity to one of protest for our rights as well as one of inclusion in who we are as individuals and as a multifaceted community. In fact, Gay Pride events must be reexamined in consideration of; whether these of celebration should instead be rallies, as was the case in the nascent days of the movement before these events were replaced by a day of partying and pride festivals drenched in commercialism.[5]

More severe still are the micro- and macroaggressions LGBTQ people are presented with every day. It's hard to come of age and come into one's own, incorporating the many identities we hold—our intersectionality—with our gay identity, when we live in fear of retaliation for simply being who we are. These aggressions undermine us and are a de facto effort on the part of society to "undignify" our lives. When discriminatory words, action, and policies are hurled at us, and when our lives are at risk, we need to muster our resources, fight for our rights, and, in doing so, embolden the dignity and pride we feel about our lives. That is why the work we must undertake individually and collectively must be more than about pride; it must be about dignity.

While sociopolitical contexts have changed in the last 50 years, the process of realizing and actualizing one's self as gay very much remains a struggle. Some 50 years after Stonewall we have also come to appreciate and respect that such challenges are even more striking for our trans peers. The psychological process of coming out is unaltered across the generations, and many of the emotions and challenges are fixed. The 15 men whose life stories constitute the heart and soul of this book speak to this fact.

On a personal note, conducting these interviews and writing this book stirred many emotions within me, including the pain I first felt when I started realizing I was gay. I would rush home crying for much of second grade, and when I came out at age 18, though I told no one but my family, I still managed to become the target of gossip in my Greek American neighborhood—idle chit-chat that served as a source of amusement in their lives. George Zafiris, my one childhood friend, stood by me. The feelings of love and friendship he had for me remained unaltered, as he adjusted his own views and knowledge to accommodate me as a young gay man. He didn't change how he cared about me. This is why this book is dedicated to him and this is why after 50 years he remains my dearest and closest friend.

Throughout this book I have sought to disentangle the similarities and differences of gay men's social, emotional, and sexual evolution during different historical periods of time; highlight the commonalties of these coming out experiences across the decades; and show that regardless of generation how gay men's lives are shaped by myriad forces—otherness and loneliness, racism, culture, class, hypermasculinity, drugs, and sex— that all seem to cut across time to some extent, telling these many stories is one small step in further owning our dignity. As gay men we are not about asking for acceptance or for normalizing our lives. In fact, we are very normal in our differences and our stories are American stories. We who have lived these stories must tell them, or our history may be lost or transformed at the hands of those who seek to homogenize and sanitize. It is only recently that we have begun to emerge from the cauldron of white straight male privileged US histories to tell the stories of many people of diverse voices. We are one of those peoples.

As gay men, and as Americans, we must be ensured lives with dignity, not struggle to achieve it as we have in the past. Our lives *are* American lives. By embedding the lives of gay men and LGBTQ people into the fabric of American society we create a world for future generations not of toler-ance or acceptance, but of complete *inclusion*. In retelling these stories, it is my hope that I have continued to add to the growing body of work that documents the beauty of our lives. I want the words shared in these pages to move our discussion forward by dispelling the stereotypes of gay men and by providing a roadmap for future generations so they can all live their lives with no second thought about whom they want to, or can, have sex with or love. If we can achieve these goals, gay men and all members of the LGBTQ community will experience the life of dignity that every human being deserves.

We seek only to live our lives with dignity and pride, as did Peter Cott and Kenneth Leedom, a couple for 58 years, who died respectively in 2014 and 2018 after decades of love and support. While the two men are a gay white couple of privilege, and do not represent the totality of the gay male experience, their story of love is nonetheless compelling and universal. According to a 2018 article by reporter John Leland, Mr. Leedom and Mr. Cott were both welcomed and embraced by each other's families, and the discussion of their gay identity never took place, as if it wasn't necessary—they were out, proud, and unapologetic.[6] These two amazing men, both born in the 1920s, were first featured in a piece by Leland in 2013,[7] when they were 89 and 88 respectively, interviewing them in what would be their last home together in a senior living facility in Lower Manhattan. They were married in a civil union ceremony in Vermont in 2000 and lived much of their life in Chelsea, which still remains a gay enclave in New York City, in a townhouse they bought for $150,000 and sold for $4,000,000.

These gay men are in fact members of the *pre*-Stonewall Generation. Undoubtedly Cott and Leedom witnessed the events that shaped the life experiences of all three generations of gay men portrayed in this book— from the Stonewall Generation to the AIDS Generation, to today's Queer Generation. In the end, as their lives came to a close, their love and their relationship was honored and revered. We can only hope that moving forward gay men like them will never have to hide who they truly are, can love each other openly and freely, without shame or fear, and remain out in and across time.

REFERENCES

1. Halkitis PN, Krause KD, Vieira DL. Mental health, psychosocial challenges and resilience in older adults living with HIV. *HIV and Aging.* 2017;42:187–203.
2. Halkitis PN. Embracing the otherness of gay men in the Trump-Pence era. *Huffington Post* 2016.
3. Harris EA. Same-sex parents still face legal complications. *New York Times* 2017.
4. Halkitis PN. Rutgers dean: why racism must be addressed within gay population | Opinion. *Newark Star Ledger* 2017.
5. Severson K. Gay Pride's choice: march in protest or dance worries away. *New York Times* 2017.
6. Leland J. An ending for a love story. *New York Times* 2018.
7. Leland J. Two men, 58 years and counting: a love story. *New York Times* 2013.

INDEX

app era, 22, 147–48
Asian men
    cultural stereotypes about, 117
    issues faced by, 140–41
    racially based "ghettoization," 139–40
    slang about, 135–36
    sociosexual politics, 139
Attitude (masculinity survey), 111, 115

Baby Boomers, 39
Baker, Gilbert, 144
Baldwin, James, 14
Barnes, Clive, 122
Beginners (film), 38
Behavioral Risk Factor Surveillance System, 87–88
Ben-Ary, Adital, 68
The Birdcage (film), 126
black LGBTQ youth, socialization of, 133
black men
    compartmentalization of, 139–40
    cultural stereotypes about, 117
    hypermasculinity and, 118–19
    objectification/dismissal of, 138
    racial preferences by, 140
    sexual racism, 141
Blank, Roman, 38
Bobby (author's husband), x, 11, 83–84, 159
Bommer, Matt, 15–16
"bottom shaming," 115
Boys in the Band (play), 15, 121–22
Brantley, Ben, 121–22
brothers, support of, 78
Bruni, Frank, 140
bullying, 86, 92–93, 113, 150, 161
BUMPS study (2005), 156
The Butch Manual (Henley), 113, 114
"butchness"/butch culture, 113, 114, 115,
    116, 120

Cain, Matt, 111
Call Me by Your Name (film), 101, 102
"Can We Please Come Up With a New Way to
    Say 'Coming Out'" (*Queerty*), 52–53
Cass, Vivienne, 4–5, 6
The Celluloid Closet (documentary), 121–22
The Celluloid Closet (Russo), xii
Center for Research and Study of the Family
    (University of Haifa), 68
Chalamet, Timothée, 101
Chee, Alexander, 139
"Chelsea Boy," 137
"chemsex," 149
childhood
    awareness of same-sex attraction, 15
    development of gay identity, 20, 53
    fantasies during, 17

feelings of otherness in, 91, 94–95
    sex education and, 160–61
    transition from, 54
class/social class. *See also* intersectional
        identities; intersectionality
    battle against AIDS and, 143
    coming out process and, 133, 167
    masculinity and, 117
    racial background and, 134
    sexual identity and, 25, 28
cohort/cohorts
    connecting across, 47
    drug use/sex risk in, 156
    fear within, 34
    P18 Cohort Study, 147–48
Cole, David D., 93
Coleman, Eli, 4–5, 56–59, 60, 64, 65. *See also*
        "Developmental Stages of the Coming-
        Out Process" model (Coleman)
coming of age
    during AIDS era, 76–77
    author's experience of, 114
    challenges of, 34–35
    drug use and, 147–48, 155–56
    feeling of otherness and, 137
    in fiction, 33
    gay identity and, 54
    gay sex and, 160
    images of gay men and, 41
    in LGBTQ community, 14–15, 48, 59
    race/ethnicity and, 142
    sexual exploration and, 60
    societal standards and, 57
coming out. *See also* age, at coming out;
        parental reaction
    author's experience of, 114
    challenges/hurdles of, 3
    as communal phenomenon, 68
    as complex/difficult, xi
    as continuous act/process, 3, 5, 52–53
    environment and, 133
    health of gay men and, xi–xii, 6
    intersectional identities and, 133–34
    to parents, 67
    pre-coming out period, 57
    as psychological process, 5
    as rite of passage, 3
    sociopolitical/cultural circumstances
        of, 56
coming out stories
    across generations, xi
    author's, ix–x
    defining experiences and, 65
    intersectionality and, 142
    retelling of, 5
    socioeconomic background and, 63